CREATING CULTURE THROUGH HEALTH LEADERSHIP

T0136913

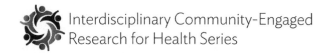 Interdisciplinary Community-Engaged
Research for Health Series

The *Interdisciplinary Community-Engaged Research for Health* series aims to bridge the gap between researchers and practitioners to facilitate the development of collaborative, equitable research and action. The reality of persistent health disparities and structural inequalities highlights the need for new strategies that are social justice-driven. Traditionally, efforts have tended to be institution-based, "expert"-focused, and silo-specific. To promote health equity, diverse stakeholders with different types of expertise need to work together to solve real-world problems. This series publishes books that recognize the importance of diverse collaboration and equip readers from a variety of backgrounds with the tools and vision to center community voice in research for action.

Series Editors:

Farrah Jacquez
University of Cincinnati

Lina Svedin
University of Utah

Advisory Board:

Sherrie Flynt Wallington
George Washington University

Jennifer Malat
University of Cincinnati

Kristin Kalsem
University of Cincinnati

Kathleen Thiede Call
University of Minnesota

Andriana Abariotes
University of Minnesota

CREATING CULTURE THROUGH HEALTH LEADERSHIP

Interdisciplinary Community-Engaged Research for Health Series

Volume 2

Edited by Lina Svedin

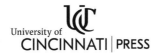
University of CINCINNATI | PRESS

About the University of Cincinnati Press

The University of Cincinnati Press is committed to publishing rigorous, peer-reviewed, leading scholarship accessibly to stimulate dialog among the academy, public intellectuals, and lay practitioners. The Press endeavors to erase disciplinary boundaries in order to cast fresh light on common problems in our global community. Building on the university's long-standing tradition of social responsibility to the citizens of Cincinnati, state of Ohio, and the world, the Press publishes books on topics that expose and resolve disparities at every level of society and have local, national, and global impact.

University of Cincinnati Press
Copyright © 2020

Published in 2020

ISBN (hardback) 978-1-947602-60-1
ISBN (e-book, PDF) 978-1-947602-61-8
ISBN (e-book, EPUB) 978-1-947602-62-5

Svedin, Lina M., editor.
Creating culture through health leadership / editor, Lina Svedin.
Interdisciplinary community engaged research for health; v. 2.
Cincinnati: University of Cincinnati Press, 2020. | Series:
   Interdisciplinary community engaged research for health; volume 2 |
   Includes bibliographical references.
LCCN 2019035407 (print) | LCCN 2019035408 (ebook) | ISBN
   9781947602601 (hardback) | ISBN 9781947602618 (pdf) | ISBN 9781947602625 (epub)
Health Promotion | Community Participation | Healthcare Disparities | Leadership
LCC RA427.8 (print) | LCC RA427.8 (ebook) | NLM WA 590 |
   DDC 362.1—dc23
LC record available at https://lccn.loc.gov/2019035407
LC ebook record available at https://lccn.loc.gov/2019035408

Designed and produced for UC Press by Jennifer Flint
Typeset in Granjon LT Std
Printed in the United States of America
First Printing

Contents

1   Leading from Within: Creating a Culture of Health
    through Leadership and Community-Grown Solutions   1
    Lina Svedin

2   Cultivating Health in Appalachia   15
    Emily Jackson

3   Saving Rural America, Starting with One Girl   29
    Michael Howard

4   Network Strategies and Cross-Collaboration
    to Strengthen Community Food Systems   47
    Tina Tamai

5   One Community, Two Voices   67
    Shannon McGuire and Jean Mutchie

6   EMBRacing Community-Engaged Research:
    Engaging, Managing, and Bonding through Race Intervention 85
    Monique C. McKenny and Riana E. Anderson

7   Rebuilding Affrilachia   111
    DeWayne Barton

8   The Evolution of Health and Housing
    for One Community-Based Organization   129
    Robert Torres

9   Building Collaboration for Community Health   149
    Lina Svedin

Bios   171

Acknowledgments   175

Index   177

CREATING CULTURE THROUGH HEALTH LEADERSHIP

Chapter 1

Leading from Within

*Creating a Culture of Health
through Leadership and Community-Grown Solutions*

Lina Svedin
University of Utah

Introduction

The stories recounted in this volume are profound illustrations and reflections on the intersectionality of health, wealth, and disparity as well as community-generated solutions to these conditions.

The chapters discuss health statuses, symptoms, and consequences in communities, in both urban and rural environments. They talk about the impacts of structural deficits and inequality, structural violence and structural racism. They talk about what that looks like, how it takes expression in families, in schools, across communities and neighborhoods, in small towns, and across mountain regions. Several stories talk about the lack of access to needed and significant healthcare. They also discuss the need for hope, skill building, leadership, and examples of how to get out of poverty and violence. The stories the authors convey tell us about the need for action, commitment, and attention to detail to teach young people, community members, and families to take action to improve their condition, to ask for what they need, to build for themselves, and to share with others.

The contributors to this volume talk about the need to be living examples of community action, organizing, and educating in order to reduce disparities in health, and increase access and community resources. They also share how they themselves served as examples and what their experiences of community organizing, building, and resourcing have been like. These culture of health leaders have built networks of people and groups that take action and create public goods to improve their own lives and that of the community in which they live.

This volume is part of a larger series of books on interdisciplinary community-engaged research for health, and this book represents a practitioner's view on community engagement and how we can build a culture of health through community-grown solutions.

The Culture of Health Leaders Program

The Robert Wood Johnson Foundation (RWJF) has been committed to improving health and healthcare for over forty years. The foundation provides county health rankings with resources for evidence-based strategies for improving health behaviors to the social determinants of health (County Health Rankings & Roadmaps 2019a) on its web page. Beyond the full report of county health rankings, there is a report called "What Works? Social and Economic Opportunities to Improve Health" (County Health Rankings & Roadmaps 2019b). It goes step-by-step into bona fide methods for improving education, social supports, health, and equity across the United States. The commitment by the foundation led to the establishment of four national programs to build a culture of health in the United States.

The Robert Wood Johnson Foundation's Culture of Health program (Culture of Health Leaders 2019) may be the most comprehensive and multifaceted method for tackling inequity in health outcomes to date. The focus on equity and working in and through communities is pivotal. That leading for health is a very hands-on, action-oriented matter is clear from resources such as "What Works for Health Disparity Rankings" and "What Works for Health" shortcut strategy adoption guides that the Culture of Health Leaders program provides. These practice-oriented resources help policymakers—among others—make decisions that, at the very least, will decrease health disparities between ethnic, racial, socioeconomic, and geographic groups.

As recipients of the RWJF's Culture of Health Leaders fellowships, the authors in this volume have received training, mentoring, and support. This program is an "opportunity for people working in every field and profession who want to use their influence to advance health and equity" to develop leadership skills. These practitioners have been trained "to collaborate and provide transformative leadership to address health equity in their communities" (Culture of Health Leaders 2019). The Culture of Health Leaders program has purposefully directed their support to include "representation from fields as diverse as business, technology, architecture, education, urban farming, the arts and many others" (Culture of Health Leaders 2019), and they seek to be ever more inclusive in terms of representation "from fields and professions across the private, public, nonprofit and social sectors to build a truly diverse group of leaders" (Culture of Health Leaders 2019). As culture of health leaders, the authors are engaging in a three-year learning experience, "including individual and team-based projects that encourage innovation, discovery, and hands-on application" (Culture of Health Leaders 2019). They work with nontraditional partners to produce "health initiatives, engage authentically with communities to change systems and institutions, and share their professional and life experiences in support of other leaders and the field" (National Collaborative for Health Equity 2019). They have, through interaction with and guidance by "nationally recognized subject matter experts, mentors, and coaches," started to "lead change within and among systems and institutions" (National Collaborative for Health Equity 2019).

Practitioners and Community Leaders Sharing to Pave the Way

The challenges to health, wellness, and health equity in the United State are massive. We face the long-term health impacts of structural racism, unequal access to education, safe housing and neighborhoods, income inequality, lack of mental healthcare and resources, multiple and repeated adverse childhood experiences, substance use disorders, high maternal and infant mortality rates, and actual declining years of life expectancy for women. We know, for instance, that "as income increases or decreases, so does health. Employment provides income that shapes choices about housing, education, child care, food, medical care, and more. Employment also often includes benefits that can support healthy lifestyle choices, such as health insurance. Unemployment and under employment limit these choices and the ability to accumulate savings and assets that can help cushion in times of economic distress" (County Health Rankings & Roadmaps 2019e).

The impact of current social determinants of health are significant and cumulative. However, as this volume showcases, we also have a growing number of hands-on ways to address the impact of these negative trends. "People with greater social support, less isolation, and greater interpersonal trust live longer and healthier lives than those who are socially isolated. Neighborhoods richer in social connections provide residents with greater access to support and resources than those that are less tightly knit" (County Health Rankings & Roadmaps 2019c). We also know now that "individuals with more education live longer, healthier lives than those with less education, and their children are more likely to thrive" and that "this is true even when factors like income are taken into account" (County Health Rankings & Roadmaps 2019d) . We have a growing set of community-fostered solutions to disparities on the ground and community-led efforts to buck the trend of worsening population health trends and address the conditions that allow inequality to fester.

Among the organizations and persons doing this work, a select group of individuals have been given the resources and training to grow as culture of health leaders. Most of the authors in the volume are deeply embedded in the communities they talk about; they are *of* the communities and *for* the communities they live and work in. Many of them have faced the adversities that they are now working to address. As practitioners, community leaders, and culture of health pioneers, they lead from within.

The work the authors exemplify and talk about is hard. That is, it is not easy to do but it is frequently simple and it can be done—and it is always, always community centered. The community-based solutions and innovations they talk about are powerful, and they show us how they did it so we can do it. These men and women share their experience as leaders doing important culture of health work to empower others to try this in their own communities. The authors' stories convey what sometimes seem like insurmountable challenges of intricate and complex situations that affect people's health and make the struggle come alive for those of us who want to change these circumstances. The authors show us how we can take steps to do that, to avoid some pitfalls they have explored and how we can utilize what they have found helpful and effective.

Methods for Community-Engaged Work

The definition of community-engaged research in the series that this volume is a part of is a collaboration between community members and researchers where resources and knowledge are exchanged through a reciprocal partnership to the benefit of both. While the core goals "of community-engaged research are action, impact, and community benefit" (Jacquez and Svedin 2020), the results are not always forthcoming. Many researchers avoid community-engaged work because it is messy and emotionally challenging. It frequently flies in the face of a clean, easily controlled, clearly measurable work process. It commonly veers away from the outlined research plan and protocol, making it far less likely to yield clear-cut results and neat stacks of statistics to be analyzed in a well-lit sterile environment. The strengths of controlled clinical trials, however, is what they add to things, such as precision medicine. There is absolutely a need for this type of clinical science, but it is not easily adapted to a community environment and open to community input.

People are doing community-engaged research in almost every academic field, but the terms assigned to describe this work vary. Some call it *action research* or *participatory action research*; others call it *civic engagement* or *community-engaged scholarship*. Others still discuss community-engaged research in terms of *consumer engagement* or *community-based participatory research* (CBPR) as they try to improve healthcare and health outcomes by partnering with those affected. What these efforts have in common is the determination to match the knowledge and methodology expertise of researchers with the local expertise and lived experiences of community members and to foster this cross-disciplinary collaboration in support of change. Community-academic partnerships may vary in their degree of collaboration—ranging from cooperation to coordination to collaboration to partnership. Each gradient of collaboration suggests more equity in leading and making decisions about the nature of the partnership and the range of activities it practices (Winer and Ray 2000).

One of the advantages of community-engaged research is that we get "the benefits of shared leadership between community and academic partners" (Jacquez and Svedin 2020), which is essential to owning the understanding of the challenges themselves as well as empowering communities to address those challenges moving forward. Even the National Institutes of Health (NIH) have underlined "the amplified impact, flow, and communication that comes with enhancing collaboration" (Jacquez and Svedin 2020) throughout the research process. Specifically, the NIH posit that shared leadership increases the potential for broader benefits in health outcomes, larger community impact, and stronger bidirectional trust built as a foundation for future collaboration.

Community-engaged research is customary in disciplines targeting a diverse set of outcomes, particularly with regards to health, but the emergence of community engagement as a key to research and impact has really taken off over the last decade. Several leading international organizations, such as the World Health Organization, now emphasize the necessity of community participation in order to accomplish population health improvements and eventually reach health equity (WHO Regional Office for Europe 2012; WHO 2016). A number of research funding organizations and mechanisms now also seem to be following this lead by requiring community-engaged research in successful grant proposals—for example, the NIH's Clinical and Translational Science Award (CTSA) program and the Patient-Centered Outcomes Research Institute (PCORI).

Working toward Change in Communities

Many people, inside and outside of visible communities, are working toward change. In this sense, we are not alone in our passion for community-engaged leadership for health. The astonishing prevalence and persistence of health inequities resulting from structural inequality in the United States is motivating researchers and institutions that fund research to pursue new ways to impact social equity across a wide variety of sectors.

Traditionally, health promotion and health improvement interventions have been institution led and "expert" driven, and address one specific aspect of health and well-being. In order to really make a dent in persistent health inequity, however, many different kinds of stakeholders need to come to the table, contributing their experience and resources. This includes, but is in no way limited to, researchers from different fields joining forces and forging their skills together for translational science. Whatever research is going to happen also needs to happen in a true partnership with community collaborators. This partnership cannot just be a connection at the top, with team leaders and directors agreeing to work together; it has to be an immersive process where those who are experiencing the inequity are respected experts and integral to the design of any research project, intervention, or possible solution.

Working in communities and across stakeholder groups and interests though collaborative processes may sound ideal, but reality too frequently places obstacles in the way of real change. Well-intentioned efforts can be derailed by a lack of funding, legislative support, organizing capacity, or compassion fatigue. Sometimes even those who work closely toward a common goal do not use the same terms to describe who they serve, what they are working toward, or what the needs of the community are. At a deeper level, stakeholders and the communities they represent can have very different goals, beliefs, and values, making their understanding of the challenges facing the community and what needs to change very different. "In order to work together toward health equity, there is a need not only to recognize the importance of collaboration but also to have the tools and vision to understand how to carry it out" (Jacquez and Svedin 2020).

Like those scholars from a wide range of disciplines who would like to engage in community-engaged research, passionate but resource-constrained practitioners have relatively few high-quality sources to turn to for methodological advice and best practices when it comes to leading and succeeding for health in communities.

The Outline of This Volume

The chapters in this volume cover the work of embedded health leaders and the communities they are working within. In chapter 2, "Cultivating Health in Appalachia," Emily Jackson explores how, as a schoolteacher, she stumbled across a startling disconnect between the children in her school and the rural land around them that grew the food they ate. This disconnect spurred Emily to start an evolving and expanding set of programs that connected schools, teachers, students, parents, and neighbors to growing and cooking fresh food. Through innovative programming Jackson showcases how she has been able to engage multiple communities in Appalachia with healthy foods and a respect for the land and people that grow the food.

In chapter 3, "Saving Rural America, Starting with One Girl," Michael Howard outlines his vision for saving rural America. Using anecdotes and examples from rural Kentucky he guides and illuminates our understanding of how social determinants of health intersect with a healthcare system in a small mining town. Far from being pessimistic, Howard uses the causal linkages between poverty, poor health outcomes, and high-cost healthcare to envision a different way of addressing healthcare needs— through community strengths, compassion, and the removal of social determinants of poor health.

In chapter 4, "Network Strategies and Cross-Collaboration to Strengthen Community Food Systems," Tina Tamai takes us to rural Hawaii and communities facing scarcity of affordable fresh fruit and vegetables. She explains how building a network of networks has increased access to fresh food and has spread education about healthy cooking and eating while honoring and preserving ethnic food culture. The work of Hawaii's Good Food Task Force and Network has been pioneering and is increasing in size and scope across the island communities.

In chapter 5, "One Community, Two Voices," Shannon McGuire and Jean Mutchie account for the development of cross-sector collaboration in order to create a culture of health in Nampa, a fast-growing city in Idaho. Their story showcases how pockets of poverty in Treasure Valley have led to significant inequality in community health status. Working with data down the census tract in Nampa, the authors identified areas of real impoverishment and lack of access to healthcare and transportation and have built a local stakeholder network to reduce childhood obesity. Through collaboration, innovation, and community engagement Nampa has managed to increase access to healthy foods and healthcare and increase mobility in an area with disproportionate rates of childhood obesity and poor health.

In chapter 6, "EMBRacing Community-Engaged Research: Engaging, Managing, and Bonding through Race Intervention," Monique McKenny and Riana Anderson recount their work with black families aimed to reduce racial stress and trauma and increase resilience among African American children. Using a positive psychological framework focused on coping skills, cultural affirmation, and strengthening parent-child relationships, the authors work to help children meet the stress of negative cultural stereotypes, discrimination, and racism that is still pervasive in the United States. By running EMBRace as a mental health and wellness intervention for African American families in West Philadelphia, McKenny and Anderson attempt to reduce the impact of racial stress and trauma on families today and in the future.

In chapter 7, "Rebuilding Affrilachia," DeWayne Barton discusses his work to rebuild Affrilachia and restore black Asheville—particularly the Burton Street neighborhood where he lives—to a healthy thriving community. Starting by picking up trash, engaging youth, and building a peace garden together with his wife, Barton has moved the community to action, rallied for space to be restored and preserved, and pulled sustainability into this community's culture. From repairing the neighborhood community center, to rallying community members young and old to fight divisive city projects, to convincing businesses to support green opportunities for youth, Barton exemplifies the extraordinary things that are possible when passionate people start doing a few simple things.

In chapter 8, "The Evolution of Health and Housing for One Community-Based Organization," Robert Torres discusses how supportive affordable housing in Boston has developed its efforts to improve health and self-sustainability among its residents. Torres's work reflects genuine commitment to building individual and community stability and sustainability. However, even with the best intentions, well-laid plans do not always work out. Their experiences include learning the importance of listening, clarifying assumptions, and working with community members to build solutions to problems they experience, and this experience was integral to Urban Edge's success story.

In chapter 9, "Building Collaboration for Community Health," Lina Svedin pulls together a set of key themes uncovered in the preceding chapters. Some of these are lessons learned and ways to forward that work. Others are reminders of issues to be taken seriously and problems that may lead to reassessment as individuals and communities work toward change. Drawing out tools and techniques that the authors and health leaders in this volume have used successfully in their communities, the concluding chapter places stepping stones on the road to community-led change.

We hope that you will be inspired and informed by the accounts of leading for health collected in this book. We bring these examples to light to serve as roadmaps for how to create a culture of health from within communities. We know that it is possible, and we hope that by reading though the authors' stories you will also be convinced.

References

County Health Rankings & Roadmaps. 2019a. "County Health Rankings." University of Wisconsin Population Health Institute in collaboration with the Robert Wood Johnson Foundation. http://www.countyhealthrankings.org/take-action-to-improve-health/what-works-for-health.

County Health Rankings & Roadmaps. 2019b. "What Works? Social and Economic Opportunities to Improve Health." Wisconsin Population Health Institute in collaboration with the Robert Wood Johnson Foundation. http://www.

countyhealthrankings.org/what-works-social-and-economic-opportunities-to
-improve-health-for-all.

County Health Rankings & Roadmaps. 2019c. "Family and Social Support." Wisconsin Population Health Institute in collaboration with the Robert Wood Johnson Foundation. https://www.countyhealthrankings.org/explore-health-rankings/measures-data-sources/county-health-rankings-model/health-factors/social-and-economic-factors/family-and-social-support.

County Health Rankings & Roadmaps. 2019d. "Education." Wisconsin Population Health Institute in collaboration with the Robert Wood Johnson Foundation. http://www.countyhealthrankings.org/explore-health-rankings/what-and-why-we-rank/health-factors/social-and-economic-factors/education.

County Health Rankings & Roadmaps. 2019e. "Income." Wisconsin Population Health Institute in collaboration with the Robert Wood Johnson Foundation. http://www.countyhealthrankings.org/explore-health-rankings/what-and-why-we-rank/health-factors/social-and-economic-factors/education.

Culture of Health Leaders. 2019. Robert Wood Johnson Foundation. http://cultureofhealth-leaders.org/about-the-program/.

Jacquez, Farrah, and Lina Svedin. 2020. "Community-Engaged Research to Improve Health and Well-Being for Young Children." In *Community-Academic Partnerships for Early Childhood Health*, edited by Farrah Jacquez and Lina Svedin, 1–20. Cincinnati, OH: University of Cincinnati Press.

National Collaborative for Health Equity. 2019. http://www.nationalcollaborative.org/our-programs/culture-of-health-leaders/.

Chapter 2

Cultivating Health in Appalachia

Emily Jackson
Appalachian Sustainable Agriculture Project

Chapter Context

As a former elementary school teacher, I saw just how disconnected children were from the source of their food and disconnected from nature in general. Wanting our next generation to have value for the natural world and to care about the food that they put in their bodies are the reasons I started the Growing Minds Farm to School program. There is so much solace that can be found in the natural world, and knowing how to grow your own food is a real-life skill. It is also a way to generate a link to our elders, as they grew up knowing about food production.

Being one of the first initiators of farm to school, I was in a position to help grow the farm-to-school movement. This meant I needed to work locally, regionally, and nationally, which was quite the stretch at certain times. Movement building is important, as most people like to belong to something and feel a kinship with others who are trying to implement this work. The development of the National Farm to School Network helped jumpstart the movement, as we could gather people together for national conferences, we had point people all across the country, and we had staff devoted to federal policy.

In this chapter I outline many lessons learned, but I will take this opportunity to elaborate on a couple. It is so important to get the adults on board for successful farm-to-school programming—you cannot effectively reach the children/students unless you have adult buy-in. At my organization, we say that kids are our low-hanging fruit … that they get it. But many adults have grown up with the taste of salt, sugar, and fat and lack necessary cooking skills (yet we blame the lack of healthy eating on children—"Oh, my kid won't eat that!"). Do not blame children for the mistakes of adults. If children are provided with experiences in the garden, cooking food they have grown, or if they have been given an opportunity to meet a local farmer/visit a local farm, then there are no problems getting the kids to try healthy food. Local food is special in that it has a face, a story, and a connection that just healthy food does not. One effective way to get teachers, administrators, and parents on board is to provide them with experiences of their own—take them on a farm field trip, conduct a taste test at a staff meeting, provide a meal of locally grown food—and you are more likely to get them involved.

Understanding the way school food works is another lesson learned that is critical to working with school nutrition staff. Take the time to understand how it works, shadow a school nutrition director, spend time talking with cafeteria managers, and then show them the respect that they deserve yet so rarely experience.

Introduction

Years ago, I was a classroom teacher in a rural community in western North Carolina. My first school was a new one, a brand-new building plunked down on land that had once been a farm. *How fitting*, I thought, *to grow a garden on this land with my students.* I imagined all the ways that I could include a garden into my instruction—the social studies, the math, the science of a garden, and the hundreds of children's books about food and farms to support language arts. Imagine my surprise when I realized that my students, though surrounded by farms and agriculture, had no idea about growing food, where food came from, or who grew it. Discussions with my students exposed yet another layer—when talking about a farm or a garden, the students spoke of their "mamaws and papaws" (grandmothers and grandfathers), not their moms and dads. My students were a generation removed from agriculture. There was a lack of connection. In 2002 I founded Growing Minds Farm to School, a program of Appalachian Sustainable Agriculture Project (ASAP), to take this idea of gardens as an instructional tool to other schools across the region. Growing Minds was born to ensure that all children understand where their food comes from, to value the land and the farmers that grow our food. Gardens also make wonderfully motivating and inspiring learning environments.

Soon this project grew to encompass more than school gardens. The program integrates edible gardens, farm field trips, and classroom cooking into the existing school curriculum. The organization also served to connect local farmers and school nutrition directors, providing locally grown food to students. At first, the work was local, creating champions of teachers and school nutrition staff, helping teachers and schools establish school gardens, connecting and growing the farm-to-school movement across western North Carolina and the southern Appalachians.

Soon after, Growing Minds connected with other organizations from across the country—thirty-plus organizations gathered at several national conferences annually and helped build what would become the National Farm to School Network. With a planning grant from the

W. K. Kellogg Foundation, ASAP and others surveyed the country about existing farm-to-school programs and came up with a body of work designed for a national farm-to-school network. In 2007 the official National Farm to School Network was launched and ASAP was selected to become the southeast regional lead agency, responsible for working in a six-state region (Kentucky, Tennessee, North Carolina, South Carolina, Georgia, and Florida).

At that time, no blueprint was available for improving how we teach about local food or connecting schools with small farmers. We were building a network from the ground up and attempting to address needs locally, regionally, and nationally. We were challenging the systems that provide food to our K–12 children. We were even challenging the US Department of Agriculture (USDA) and how they governed school nutrition services.

Local relationships taught us an important lesson—that school nutrition was doing the best they could with very little. We began to realize how little cafeteria staff was paid, how little value was placed on their work, how little money is allocated to school food, and how few people understood the way that the National School Lunch Program operates and is funded. We gauged that if we could make our communities understand how the budgets worked for school cafeterias, then parents and community members would become partners with, and advocates for, school nutrition staff. Our tactic was to become a cheerleader for school nutrition staff.

While other farm-to-school organizations began their work on local procurement, Growing Minds (ASAP) paused to consider the market opportunity that schools provided for small farmers, priding itself on matching farmers to the most lucrative markets available. K–12 schools—and, later, preschools—certainly did not fit that description. Many of the groups that began farm-to-school work came from health fields, with little to no experience dealing with local farms and helping farms become economically sustainable. For the health-focused organizations, getting locally grown food into school cafeterias clearly benefitted children and that was enough. ASAP chose a different tactic and became the farm-to-school program that lifted the educational components of farm to school (classroom cooking, edible gardens, farm field trips, cafeteria taste tests).

As the local food and farm-to-school movement grew, so did demand for programming and training. ASAP was able to attract many wonderful individuals who desired to work in this field and with Growing Minds. Through these networks, ASAP/Growing Minds quickly expanded. The Growing Minds staff of ASAP put extensive work into creating the resources and support to keep farm-to-school programming alive and growing, as evidenced by the popularity and use of our website and requests for training. Children and the larger school community needed experiences that would help them make connections that would create a demand for fresh, healthy, tasty, locally grown food. The educational components allowed us to work with a wide variety of people—chefs, parents, Cooperative Extension, farmers, university students and professors, and dietetic interns.

We spent time trying to make farm to school as easy as possible by focusing on the educational components, such as creating lesson plans that aligned with state and national competencies; free seeds and mini grants; training for teachers, farmers, school nutrition staff, community members, and Cooperative Extension. All of the activities were designed to address the barriers teachers and school nutrition services might face. Some other strategies included giving a Community Supported Agriculture (CSA) share to school nutrition staff and taking them on a field trip to the CSA farm, providing a farm-to-school conference for

Cooperative Extension agents in a three-state area, convening a meeting between school nutrition directors and area produce distributors, conducting cafeteria taste tests and demonstrating how incredibly inexpensive it could be, and providing promotional materials ("I tried local ___" stickers and recipe cards, which aligned with our lesson plans). ASAP/Growing Minds began training chefs and connecting them with teachers/classrooms long before former First Lady Michelle Obama and the Chefs Move to Schools programs brought awareness to this movement.

Getting a Head Start

In 2007 ASAP was approached by a local Head Start agency interested in procuring locally grown food directly. Despite not having a firm understanding of the early education realm, we jumped in. What a learning curve! Our partnership with Head Start resulted in us helping to establish an edible garden, connecting them with a local farmer, providing training for the Head Start staff, and, most importantly, beginning a relationship in the early childhood world. We began to realize just how important working with early childhood education could be—children were forming their attitudes and behaviors about food, and early childhood is the time that provides the best opportunity to work with parents and families and find ways to engage them in the health and education of their children.

Just as we discovered how little value is placed on cafeteria workers in the K–12 arena, we found that there is little respect for early childhood staff. Often referred to as *babysitters* or *daycare workers*, early childhood staff were underpaid and definitely not regarded as professionals. Forty-six percent of early childhood workers were part of families enrolled in at least one public safety net program, compared with

26 percent of those in the broader workforce. These very same people are responsible for the most important time in a child's life—in the first few years of life, more than one million new neural connections are formed every second. By the age of five, 90 percent of a child's brain is developed. Another mission: help lift up issues pertaining to childcare workers' salaries and the importance of the early years.

As with K–12 farm to school, building a network to grow the movement, we embarked on a similar route for early childhood by building a network to grow the movement, partnering with North Carolina Child and Adult Food Program (and others), we created the NC Farm to Preschool Network. More and more preschools, in North Carolina and other states, are offering farm-to-preschool programming to their children, based on this model.

Taking Work Upstream

Taking a strategic and systemic course, with an eye to sustaining farm-to-school efforts, ASAP and project partners took farm to school "upstream," integrating local food and farm to school into university undergraduate and graduate dietetics, nutrition, and education majors' coursework. The growing movement needed individuals whose career paths would most align with farm to school as its future champions. Rather than rely on teachers and school nutrition staff already in the field, why not energize a new generation of teachers and health professionals by engaging them in hands-on local food and farm-to-school experiences? The initiative was named Growing Minds @ University (GM@U).

Western Carolina University was the first university we approached, and today Growing Minds @ Western Carolina University serves as a model. It provides local food and farm-to-school experiences for their university students as they interact with K–12 students through cafeteria taste tests, edible garden activities, and classroom cooking. GM@U branched out to include the dietetic intern programs of Appalachian State University and Lenoir-Rhyne University. ASAP's most recent GM@U expansion was into the early childhood program at Blue Ridge Community College, integrating local food and farm to preschool into the early childhood educator program, with an end goal of including all the community colleges in the state.

In August 2018, ASAP, in partnership with Duke University's World Food Policy Center and the University of North Carolina at Chapel Hill Center for Health Promotion and Disease Prevention, hosted the "Healthy Eating in Practice" conference. Using the upstream approach from our Growing Minds @ University project, the conference targeted physicians and the healthcare industry to understand their level of influence and how that influence could be used to create healthy food environments. "Healthy Eating in Practice" provided hands-on education for practitioners, researchers, and influencers focused on changing the culture of healthcare to better support healthy eating behaviors and help prevent chronic diet-related diseases in children and families. Over three hundred individuals from thirty-two states attended. Results from conference evaluations indicate that attendees appreciated the innovative approaches—such as cooking classes and farm field trips—that showcased the various ways that healthy eating could be put into practice.

Lessons Learned along the Way

After sixteen years of programming, Growing Minds has gained a lot of experience to share with others, such as:

Lack of Connection

Children in rural areas generally had little to no knowledge of or experience with farms and food. Colleagues around the country report the same situations in their region. Children in urban areas are often assumed to have a similar lack of connection, but I would say this—at least there is a reason that urban children don't know food and farms—they live in a city! Unfortunately it's not just children who don't know where their food comes from or how it grows (recently a teacher asked me if I had apple seeds). Adults—many of whom have grown up worshipping the holy trinity of fat, sugar, and salt, and who don't necessarily know how to cook or how to grow a garden—these are the individuals who lack the knowledge and resources to make this reconnection as well, in order to model to their children healthier choices and skills with the food they buy, grow, cook, and consume.

Funding

Another example that illustrates the lack of connection is the belief that a grant or significant funding is needed in order to establish a school garden. When individuals grow gardens in their backyards, they don't seek grant funding, so why should school gardens be any different? School gardens are a wonderful opportunity to engage the community for resources to support a school garden—grandparents and/or local farmers can supply knowledge and experience, families can donate various garden tools, local nurseries and farms can supply plants … you get the picture. What are we teaching our children about gardens? That it takes a lot of money to grow a garden? The best outcome of a school garden is that the child is so excited about it that they endeavor to create one at home. Can a child do this if they think it requires lots of money and special equipment to do so? No, you just need a little land (or some containers), seeds, plants, water … easy peasy. The takeaway is that adults need to be connected to local food and farms, not just children. In fact, if adults aren't behind the program, it won't be as successful in reaching the children.

Personal before Professional

The first professor to come on board with GM@U did so because she knew it would be an intriguing and worthwhile experience for her university students. This same professor found herself becoming teary-eyed while driving to Shelton Farms one Saturday morning for a farm-to-school training session. She had recently purchased a CSA share from Shelton Farms but had never visited the farm before. She realized that she was going to see the place where her family's food came from! Initially it was the concept of the initiative that appealed to her, but, more importantly, it also had personal significance. Other professors who participated in the project were similarly attracted in a personal and professional manner, as they had moved to western North Carolina for the beauty of the mountain region and knew that farms greatly contributed to that beauty. Initiatives that have a connection to our personal lives are strong motivators and can play a part in the sustainability of the work. The lesson here is one of experiences and stories. Good candidate schools or communities need to connect with the project personally. To help them connect, ASAP helped individuals to build their own stories, by taking cafeteria staff on farm field trips, purchasing CSA shares for teachers, and bringing locally grown food products to staff meetings, which led to more success in school and community advocacy and active participation.

Education versus Health

To integrate into existing programs and curricula, as well as to honor teachers and their time, ASAP framed farm to school as a way to teach the common course of study. It is important to communicate where you are coming from when you work with schools and to be upfront about it. Admittedly, there was an outlay of extra time required up front (to establish the garden, get administrators on board, recruit volunteers, etc.). Teachers do care if their children eat healthy diets, but they must prepare their students academically. But, once teachers saw all the opportunities to integrate gardens, cooking, and farm field trips into their curriculum, there were endless opportunities for instruction, and it was a motivating experience for children. The goal of the integrated method was not only to teach children how to read, write, and do math, but to apply those skills in the garden and farm-to-school setting, where those skills could be practically applied while gardening, cooking, and learning about food and health.

Procurement versus Education

Schools and preschools are not the best market opportunity for farmers, especially if they have access to more lucrative ones. However, not all farmers have access to the lucrative markets and all communities have schools, so it can be a good match in certain situations. Selling food to schools can also be part of a farm's market diversification or it can be a good stepping stone to working with other institutional buyers (hospitals, universities, etc.). The educational components of farm to school—school gardens, classroom cooking, cafeteria taste tests, and farm field trips—all help children (and adults) make connections to local food and farms.

Farm to school is hands-on, is centered on the students' experiences, and can be integrated into the existing curriculum as well as meaningfully involve the larger school community. Farmers can play a large role in hosting students on farm field trips, assisting with school gardens, and providing local food for cafeteria taste tests. The educational components are the best place to start—get children and adults excited about healthy, locally grown food, before investing a lot of hard work toward getting that local product procured for the entire school system. I will never forget the conversation I had with one of my students. As he was eating a raw beet in the garden, Jesse asked why our school didn't serve beets in the cafeteria. Would he have asked that question if he hadn't grown the beet himself?

Working within Existing Systems

After successfully establishing a school garden or implementing cafeteria taste tests, the next step could be to work with school nutrition staff to procure locally grown food and champion nutrition. It is hard work to understand how school food works (that's an entire chapter in and of itself). To reduce the start-up hurdles, consider making local procurement as easy as possible. In schools that are self-operated, the district is already purchasing their produce from a produce distributor. Follow the lead of ASAP by working with local distributors to connect them with local growers, to source locally grown food into their distribution. This strategy allows the school nutrition staff to continue working with a known entity (sometimes referred to as an approved vendor) and get their local and their nonlocal produce from one source. Getting local produce into an existing distributor's system can also result in helping to provide local food products for the other customers of that produce company. Some schools are willing to work directly with local growers, but there is a limit to how many they can manage directly. Getting local farmers' food into the produce distributor's offerings makes it easier for both the farmer and the school nutrition staff. For example, there are forty-one schools in Buncombe County, North Carolina. Not many farmers are equipped (or desire) to distribute to so many schools. Produce distributors, on the other hand, have the capacity, infrastructure, knowledge, and experience to work with entire school systems.

Conclusion

If you had asked me ten years ago about the number of organizations involved in farm to school in the Southeast, I could have rattled off not only the numbers but the people involved. Today, I couldn't begin to do that. The movement has grown so fast and appeals to such a wide variety of players, that now all fifty states have some type of farm-to-school programming. Statewide coalitions, state agency staff whose full-time jobs are farm to school, and numerous farm-to-school policy initiatives (at the local, state, and national levels) all exist. Now an ever-growing variety of creative and impactful ways to approach farm to school/preschool are available for those who wish to build or improve their local programs.

Chapter 3

Saving Rural America, Starting with One Girl

Michael Howard
Baptist Health Madisonville

Chapter Context

I grew up in a small town in rural western Kentucky. Unlike most of my friends, I loved growing up there. Most of them couldn't wait to shake off the dust, get out, and never come back. If I could have done the things I wanted to do there, I would have never left. But I did have to leave, and pursued a career in academia for over twenty years. I did, however, try to plant some seeds that might allow me to come home one day. Some ten years after planting, the seeds sprouted and a completely unexpected opportunity to come home arose. By that time, I was settled elsewhere and found it difficult to take the opportunity. I interviewed for the position three times without accepting. After the third interview, the president of the hospital called me and said, "I don't know what else to tell you, but if you take this job, you'll be in a position to impact the health of the people in your hometown." That was something I could get behind, so I took the job.

My interest in healthcare administration was not particularly consuming, but the part of the job that allowed me to work in community health and with medical learners in our education programs was great. The more I studied and learned about rural community health and wellness, the more I realized that rural communities are much more fragile than urban ones. Many small communities have practically collapsed after the loss of their primary employer. The brain drain of talented youth is a huge loss to rural places. Poverty and poor health are more prevalent. There is rarely any tradition of wellness or healthy culture. Resources are usually pretty limited in terms of community action and support. The thing is, in rural communities, all of these factors are directly connected. You can't really move the needle by working on one thing. In rural communities, you have to dig down to find the root causes of issues and then you have to bring all available resources to bear on them in order to make a lasting difference. Otherwise, you are just continually working to react to the consequences of deeper, more complex problems. I want to help fix my hometown and aid it and its people along to a healthier, more prosperous future.

Rural communities have to make the most of the resources that they have. There just aren't enough funds, people, time, and will to waste any of it on activities that don't change the fundamental issues. My project is to pull together all those stakeholders into a broad-based coalition to collectively identify and address the fundamental issues affecting individuals, families, and the community at large. Coalition building is a tested and effective mechanism to make differences, particularly in rural communities. If we can bring together the healthcare providers, the social service providers, the housing people, the nutrition people, the transportation people, the governmental entities, and the community leaders to plan, gather data, develop long-term unified strategic visions, and act collectively to achieve the outcomes we have identified, we will change the trajectory of this community and, by example, other rural communities that are facing similar challenges.

We are still working on this project and will be for many years. We are attempting to change culture, both among the citizens of the community and the organizations and community leaders who are doing the work. Culture change takes time. One thing I've learned is that there is a great deal of inertia in rural communities. People don't like change. Helping people to understand the need for change is hard. Getting them to actually do anything to change is even harder. Another lesson is that rural communities have something of an inferiority complex. There is a tendency for people to believe that issues are "too big" and that "we can't do that here." It is difficult to even get community leaders to buy into the possibilities. The failure of vision is probably the most common reason rural communities can't break free from the baggage of the past while still maintaining the positive aspects of rural life.

Introduction

The ultimate goal of our project is to save rural America. I've never had any problem dreaming big. It's a lofty goal, to be sure, but a worthy one. The good news is that there are a number of intermediate goals that will be beneficial as well, just in case we don't get all the way to that grand prize, but I really do think it is possible.

I was born in the best town on earth. At least that was what the great big, blue signs that spanned the main roads into town said, "Welcome to Madisonville, Kentucky, the Best Town on Earth." As far as I could tell when I was a youngster, it was true. I had a good family, safely ensconced in the middle class, and small-town life agreed with me. My dad was the administrator of the local tuberculosis hospital and my mom was a nursing instructor. Madisonville was quite the prosperous little town back then, thanks to one of the other informational offerings on the big, blue signs that said, "Heart of the Coalfield." Madisonville is located pretty much smack in the middle of what was called the western Kentucky coalfield, which was then, and had been, off and on for some time, the largest coal-producing area of the United States. This last bit is very central to the story. It is, directly and indirectly, why I came back home, why we're trying to build a new culture of community health, and why it can actually work, despite the fact that we're in the rural south, which, as everyone knows, is not the most amenable place to pursue change.

Coal Mining in Madisonville

Madisonville sits on what was, about three hundred million years ago, an enormous swamp. As the trees, ferns, vines, and other plants died and fell into the water, they began to decay. Eventually the layer of dead plant material was covered up by silt, cutting the mat of dead plant matter off from the oxygen in the air. Over millennia, the plant material turned first to peat, and then with increasing pressure and heat build-up, the peat slowly turned to lignite (a type of low-quality brown coal), then to sub-bituminous coal (which is still rather soft), then to the hard, black, energy-dense, bituminous coal that has been mined around here for about 150 years. My grandfather was an electrician in the mines until he died of a heart attack at the age of fifty-nine. My brother-in-law retired from the mines in 2015. Even though most of the mines have long since shut down, there are few people from this area who didn't either work in the mines or have family who did.

Healthcare in Madisonville

This mining history is significant for a couple of reasons. First, coal mines, at least since the end of World War II, paid well, leading most industries in the area of employer-provided healthcare. So, we had a lot of families around here with good health insurance plans. What we didn't have was enough physicians in the area to care for the population. In 1948 Dr. Loman Trover completed his medical training and set up a practice in his hometown of Earlington, Kentucky, a small mining town just south of Madisonville. In 1950 his brother, Faull, joined his brother and they established a new practice in Madisonville. These two brothers, particularly Loman, recognized two things. They recognized that medicine was changing from the old general practitioner/solo practice model to a more sophisticated model employing specialists of all disciplines. They also recognized that Madisonville, being in the heart of the coalfield that employed thousands of coal miners with excellent health insurance, was a great place to build a medical center. And build it they did.

The Trover Clinic was established and moved into its first facility in 1952. In 1953 the Trover brothers recruited their first partner, to practice orthopedics. Then they brought on a cardiologist. Then they brought aboard a general surgeon. By 1958 the practice had expanded to sixteen physicians. The county hospital, built by the New Deal Works Progress Administration in 1938, had fifty-four beds that were, by the late 1950s, becoming insufficient. Over the years, the Trover Clinic expanded—building new buildings, building satellite clinics in towns throughout the region, which required the hospital to expand. The hospital expanded to 121 beds in 1959, then to 179 in 1962. By 1965 there were thirty-four physicians in the medical group, covering most of the specialties of the time. In 1969 the hospital expanded again, to 272 beds. Ultimately the practice would, by the early 1980s, include over one hundred physicians and became the biggest group medical practice in Kentucky. A new, 410-bed hospital was completed in 1979 to accommodate the needs of a growing patient population. To have a medical infrastructure of this size and sophistication is unusual outside of a large urban center, and to have it in a town of seventeen thousand people in rural western Kentucky is pretty unique.

The Issue

The second reason the history of coal mining in this area is significant to my story is that the mines pretty much are history, now. Coal production peaked around 1990, but mine employment actually peaked right after World War II. Automation and better machinery cut mine employment by about half in the 1950s, and employment slowly increased with increased production up until about 1990 but never reaching near the numbers employed in the late 1940s to early 1950s. Coal production now is about half what it once was in the area, and there are only two mines still working in the county, directly employing fewer than 850 people. It is the story of much of rural America. What is a company town supposed to do when the company shuts down? People don't build towns for no reason. Every town was built because there was a port, factory, market, railroad, or something there to give people a reason to build a town. Some of those towns take off and grow into cities, but most just stay small towns. People open shops and ancillary businesses, but the town stays centered on the primary economic engine. Young people who don't see their futures tied to that industry leave and they usually don't come back. Then things change and, suddenly, there is a town with no real reason to exist anymore, just like Madisonville.

So, to set the stage, here we have a small coal-mining town where the mines are mostly gone. However, that history has left a legacy that endures. First is the existence of our medical center, which is still remarkable in scope and capacity for a rural area. To service the mines and the medical center back in the day, large numbers of professionals were drawn to the area. Medical professionals, engineers, lawyers, business people, and others came to the area, generating a good bit of economic activity, but also demanding such amenities as good schools, public works, and community amenities while also supporting community services and organizations. Significant fortunes were made by some people from the coal industry, the medical center, and various associated businesses, and some of those families still live in the area, representing a significant amount of realized and potential philanthropy.

It is the hospital now, and not mining, that is the economic engine of the county, both in terms of employees and payroll. The schools are still good, ranking in the top quartile in the state. We have a large number of active and effective community service organizations, and a good deal of community involvement and community benefit activity. Many good people live here.

If you take all of those factors together, what it all adds up to is a community that, like most of rural America, is struggling, but one that also has a great deal of potential. All the ingredients are there for something special to be done in rural western Kentucky. So, when I was given an opportunity to come home, I took it, with one overarching goal—to try to help make Madisonville and western Kentucky into an example of what rural communities in their second acts can become in a world and a time where resources and power are becoming ever more centralized in urban areas. If it can be done anywhere, we should be able to do it here. We may not be able to get all the way to the "Best Town on Earth," but maybe we can get close. For sure, we can build a much brighter future for everyone.

Which leaves two questions: What are we going to do? And how are we going to do it?

Rural Kentucky's Health Challenges

We're not proposing anything new or revolutionary in Hopkins County. Most of what we are going for has already been tried in other places and has been shown to be effective in improving health for individuals and families. There is no need to reinvent the wheel. We're just taking a number of good ideas and adapting them to our place, our time, and our goals.

The medical center in Madisonville may be unusual in size and capability, but like most medical centers everywhere in the United States, we aren't doing it right. We still largely wait for people to get sick and then take care of them when they come to us. This "fee-for-service" model of "sick care" is what has developed mostly over the past sixty or seventy years in the United States as medicine has become more sophisticated, complicated, and technological. Diagnosing and treating illness often requires a great deal of complex, heinously expensive equipment and highly trained people to operate it. The only way to do that is to bring people to a central location where all those resources can be efficiently concentrated. There are a number of benefits and drawbacks to this system. The main benefit is probably the extent to which diseases can be treated. The modern medical center has an incredible ability to identify and treat sickness, thanks to all that advanced technology and medical expertise. The main drawback is that it is expensive. Very expensive.

For all the money we spend on healthcare, as a nation, we aren't very healthy. Western Kentucky is a particularly unhealthy part of a very unhealthy state. Our longevity and quality of life are low. Our rates of diabetes, heart disease, pulmonary disease, and cancer are much higher than national averages. Our rates of smoking, adult and childhood obesity, physical inactivity, poor nutrition, and poverty are also well above national averages. Most of our health metrics are also trending in the wrong direction—our health is, in many ways, getting worse over time, not better. In 2018 the average lifespan in the United States decreased from the previous year for the third year in a row. A significant contributor to that worrying trend is the increase in deaths from opioid-related overdoses. The Appalachian region of eastern Kentucky has been the hardest-hit part of the country by the opioid epidemic. Fortunately, as of late 2018, western Kentucky has been largely spared by the drug crisis, but our overdose deaths are inching upward.

While the sharp rise in opioid-related deaths has impacted the national lifespan, it isn't the only factor. We are just becoming unhealthier over time. There have been many studies seeking to identify why this is so and what can be done about it. These studies agree that healthcare, as we typically define it, plays only a relatively small roll in overall health—perhaps about 20 percent. The other 80 percent of the factors that influence health are socioeconomic in nature. How and where we live plays a large role. The choices we make—in terms of what we eat, how (or if) we exercise, whether or not we smoke—all play a huge role. One of the biggest contributors to poor health is poverty. Collectively, these factors are called the social determinants of health, and they are the primary factors in determining how healthy a person is likely to be and how long they are likely to live. In fact, the factor that is most closely correlated to how long a person is likely to live is not genetics, education, or income. It is the zip code they lived in when they were born.

Trends in Healthcare

Okay. Now we know that medical care only accounts for about 20 percent of health. What do we do about it? There are lots of things, some of which are obvious and easy, some of which aren't. One big driver of change is going to come from entities that pay for healthcare. There are three main groups of people, regarding how healthcare is paid for: people with private insurance, people with public insurance, and people with no insurance. The world of healthcare finance in the United States is an incredibly complex place, but no matter who is paying the bills, they would prefer to pay as little for it as possible. The federal government, through the Center for Medicare and Medicaid Services (CMS), is by far the largest payer, and plays a very outsize role in determining what standards of care are and how much providers are going to be paid to provide care.

Recognizing that our fee-for-service model is unsustainable, CMS has determined that we are going to transition to another system called value-based healthcare. In the new model, providers will be paid a certain amount to keep their patients healthy, and more or less be penalized for when their patients have a preventable hospitalization. The idea is that it will cost much less to help people stay healthy than to fix them when they get sick. Private payers have also recognized this and have begun promoting primary care delivery models, such as the patient-centered medical home (PCMH), that are similarly designed to provide well care instead of sick care. That's all very well and good, but the question remains: what are we going to do about it?

Identifying the Root of the Problem

That's where our coalition comes in. If the current medical infrastructure isn't the answer to building healthier communities, what is? Say, for instance, that we have a twelve-year-old girl who comes into our emergency room (ER) eight or ten times a year with an acute asthma attack. This is fairly easy to treat, so we take care of her attack and send her home, knowing full well that we will be seeing her again in a month, or so. Her ER visit probably cost a couple of thousand dollars, some of which will be paid for by Medicare, with the rest being written off by the hospital. She's going to be back because her home is full of black mold, which exacerbates her asthma. Her home is full of black mold because the pipes under the kitchen sink leak. What this girl needs most to take care of her asthma is a plumber, not a doctor. So, is it leaky pipes that are at the root of her health problems? Would fixing the leaks take care of the situation? Let's examine the situation a little deeper.

Why are the pipes leaking? Well, the pipes have been leaking because her mom can't afford to get someone to fix them. Why can't she afford to get someone to fix them? Because she works two jobs, but they are both low paying, so that still doesn't leave enough money to pay a plumber. Why can't she get a better job? She has no job skills. Why doesn't she have any job skills? She's tried a couple of job training programs, but she hasn't completed either one. Why hasn't she completed a program? Because she has a substance use disorder (SUD). Why does she have a SUD? Because she got in a car wreck three years ago and got addicted to prescription pain medication.

What the little girl with the asthma problem actually needs the most to be healthy isn't a doctor, or even a plumber. What the little girl needs is substance abuse treatment for her mother. If her mom gets through that, then she can get some job skills, get a job that pays a living wage so she can pay her own plumber. Then the mold goes away, the asthma attacks stop (mostly), and the little girl and her mother start living a normal life.

There are, as you might imagine, a number of implications here. The biggest one is that the solution to what first manifests as a medical issue is very often to be found outside the hospital or the clinic. It is to be found in the streets and in people's homes—in their choices or lack thereof. Poverty is often a player, but not always. Making a person, a family, or a community healthier is usually much more about socioeconomics and demographics than it is about genetics or physiology.

Most communities have the resources to deal with many of the issues being faced by the family in our story. There are social service agencies. There are housing authorities. There are SUD treatment centers. There are job training centers. There are all sorts of public and private charitable organizations. And there are hospitals. For the purposes of our story, let's assume that the community she lives in has a wide range of active community service and support organizations. So why does our girl still end up in the ER with acute asthma every month or so? The answer to that is the same as the answer to questions such as: "Why are many urban school districts underperforming?" or "Why has the poverty rate held more-or-less steady for the past fifty years?" Trillions of dollars have been spent since the war on poverty began in 1964. Why haven't we won? Why are our people no healthier? Why are the achievement gaps still so wide in schools?

The reason is something I discovered (though other people have known it for ages) about five years ago when I was still a faculty member at an urban university. I walked into a meeting about "service learning," which was something I knew nothing about at the time, although it sounded like something I would like to incorporate into my classes. I still don't know much about service learning, but that meeting was transformative for me on a number of different levels. Present were two administrators from the failing urban K–12 school district in which our university was located. There were also a couple of faculty members from our College of Education and me. The main thrust of this meeting was that our education faculty wanted to work on a program with the school district to provide assistance to their STEM (Science, Technology, Engineering, and Math) teachers, because their student outcomes for those classes were horrifically bad, beginning in elementary school and carrying through, as you might imagine, to middle school. We got to talking about things that the schools needed. One of the administrators told me that one of his big wishes was to introduce more citizenship activities into the elementary and middle schools. I was a Scout leader at the time, so I asked if they had Cub Scouts in their schools. He said they tried every now and again to start up a troop, but they inevitably failed after a year or two, due to lack of adult participation. You need to understand at this point how truly clueless I was to issues like this. I really had no conception of the factors in play in this area. So, I asked, "Why?"

The guy explained that the parents who were the ones who tried to do things like that were also the parents working two or three jobs to try to make ends meet. At some point, they would just run out of time to spend on Scouts, since they were spending all their time trying to make a living. This hit me pretty hard. We then got into a discussion about the abysmal state of the district's finances. One of the administrators mentioned how expensive it was to keep their school buildings open all year. I asked, in my ignorance, why they kept them open. He said they kept them open because many of their students only get to eat when they are at school, so they keep the buildings open so the free breakfast and lunch program can stay active. Wow. My world view took a big hit at that time. Then we get to talking about their science classes. One big problem, of many, according to the school administrator was that the class rosters were very fluid, so it was extremely difficult to know at which level any particular student was at any point in time. I once again asked, "Why?" Well, the administrator told me, many of their students are functionally homeless, couch surfing with their families at various friends' and relatives' houses or moving from one apartment with free first month's rent to another. As they moved around, they switched schools or even districts. By this time, I was practically in a puddle on the floor. Of course these kids aren't doing well in their STEM classes. It's pretty hard to worry about photosynthesis when you don't know where you're going to sleep that night or whether or not you'll get to eat dinner. This was when I realized that the problem with these schools wasn't the teachers. It wasn't the facilities. The biggest issues for these schools weren't even in the buildings at all. It was in the neighborhoods and the streets and the homes. You can throw money at the schools all day long, but new buildings or more computers aren't going to fix the problem. Scared, hungry kids aren't going to learn much in school. The real problem doesn't lie where it would seem to. This certainly isn't news to a lot of people, but it was a revelation to me. My comfortable world view was completely remodeled. Better late than never, I guess.

When I moved into healthcare, one of the first things I discovered as I started to dig into the community health literature was that many of the problems with community health are really the same as they are for urban schools. People aren't unhealthy just because of microbes or genetics (usually). They are unhealthy because of how and where they live. Trying to fix healthcare by tweaking what goes on in hospitals and clinics is the same as trying to fix education in an urban school district by buying more computers. The real issues lay somewhere else, and they usually, but not always, have some relation to poverty.

In our decades-long wars on poverty, disease, drugs, and failing schools, we have spent trillions of dollars on the wrong things. The issues we have been trying to address are only symptoms and consequences of deeper, harder-to-find root causes. New whiteboards aren't going to fix the problems in those science classrooms. Our girl's asthma won't be fixed by spending money in the emergency room. It will be helped by spending money (a lot less money, in this case) on a plumber, but until we get mom some help with her substance problems so she can start down the path to standing on her own, we will never stop those asthma attacks for good.

Our community and social services organizations are designed to work in specific areas—healthcare, food security, housing assistance, education, transportation, etc. They generally do wonderful things, applying the (usually scanty) resources they have to help address specific needs. For instance, we have a magnificent charitable organization here that raises money to buy a new pair of nice shoes for schoolkids throughout the county who need them. It fulfills a great physical and emotional need for the children. It's another one of those things I never gave much thought to, but what some of these kids wear to school would break your heart. The work that this organization does is an unalloyed good. No doubt about that. The thing is, after you buy a first-grader a pair of shoes, chances are pretty good that you're going to buy a slightly bigger pair of shoes for that same kid eleven more times by the time they graduate high school because their needing shoes is a consequence of some weightier, more complex issue that shoes alone won't fix.

Our Solution

What we propose to do in western Kentucky is simplicity itself in conception and maybe a little more complex in execution. The basic premise is that we can substantially improve the health, quality of life, and prosperity of individuals, families, and communities in the region, using existing community resources, but in a more coordinated way. The effectiveness of coalitions in community work is well documented. Like most community health coalitions, we will begin by working together to raise awareness of health issues in the public, improve access to health-related resources for all, and promote sound public policy to support health and wellness. There are hundreds of projects of this nature that have been successful in other places.

Phase 1

We're in phase 1 right now, which is where we are building the depth and breadth of our coalition, starting to educate and engage with the public, and extending our reach out into the parts of our geography and our society that don't, for one reason or another, interact with the resources that can help them live better. We're conducting health fairs, doing health screenings, gathering information from the public and from all sorts of resources to determine where our health issues are, what the public perceptions are, and how to develop strategies to address them. We're reaching out to places where people gather, trying to start a conversation that includes individual and community health. Two main categories of such places in rural communities are churches and barber/beauty shops. Lots of people in rural communities who don't go anywhere else go to church every week and become, at least briefly, part of a caring, supportive community. Most folks get their hair cut, at least occasionally. When people are at the barber shop/salon, they tend to chat. Why not chat a bit about the value of getting a blood pressure check in between discussions of why the Kentucky football/basketball team is/is not playing well. The barber/beauty shop idea is not original, but it has been shown to be effective at reaching hard-to-reach people and maybe starting a community-wide conversation. We talk to the civic clubs. We write articles for the local paper. We are building a social media presence. If we are to get anywhere in the communities in which we live, we have to develop a presence. Rural communities work like that. Change comes from inside, not outside. Relationships and trust must be built. That's mostly what we are working on now. It's like building the foundation of a house: if you don't do it well, the result won't be pretty.

Phase 2

While we are pouring the concrete on which we will build the future of our communities, we are also working on the strategy and laying the groundwork for phase 2, which is where real change will be found. Think back to our girl with asthma. If we keep doing things like we are, she's just going to keep coming back. The people in the ER will likely never know about the mold problem. They will just keep dealing with asthma. The people in the Family Resource Center at her school may know about the mold, but they aren't likely to tell the hospital about it, even if a clear mechanism to make that communication were possible. They might contact a local community organization who could help fix the pipes, but that still won't fix the problem, because there isn't enough money in the household to keep it healthy. Maybe someone will talk to her mother about career training, but if she is still fighting her addiction to her prescription meds, that's not going to take. Many organizations may be working to help, using limited resources, to ameliorate this issue or that, but until all those organizations sit down together, develop an integrated plan, and work in a coordinated, holistic fashion to address the fundamental, root cause of dysfunction in this family, none of it will work, long term. What we are doing is developing the resources to make that coordinated assault on what is making this family sick and, by association, making our community weaker.

Conclusion

Through the use of a community health coordinator, we are bringing the needed resources to bear, reducing the obstacles to accessing those resources, and providing oversight and support to make sure that what is needed is done. If the true root cause of our girl's asthma is her mom's SUD, then we have to fix the SUD. As anyone knows, that is often an extremely long, arduous process that may fail many times before it takes. All of the other things afflicting the family will still be going on, so we still have to tend to all that, but if we marshal the resources, develop a sound plan, and execute it with patience and dedication, in time what we will have is a functional family. Our girl won't end up in the ER anymore. That is good. The ER won't be writing off the cost of her care every month or so. That's good too. Mom will be able to get some training and get a job. She will then be able to pay for her own needs. Her home becomes somewhere where it is possible for a child to grow up healthy and reach her potential. Maybe she becomes the first person in her family to go to college. Maybe she becomes a nurse's aide. Or a bookkeeper. Maybe her child becomes a doctor or an engineer. The point is that this family has the chance to be healthy—physically, mentally, and socially. They become producers. The community no longer has to spend resources to manage the consequences of their situation. Most of all, the unrealized human potential is unleashed to the benefit of all.

Then we move to the next family. And the next. It is not the work of a few years or even a few decades. It is the work of generations, but with every successful intervention, people get better and stronger. Families get better. Communities get healthier. Healthier communities are more vital, more vigorous, more resilient, more adaptable, more dynamic, and more attractive. If we fix the girl's asthma, we can fix rural America. It's just a matter of will and resources. And a little time.

Chapter 4

Network Strategies and Cross-Collaboration to Strengthen Community Food Systems

Tina Tamai
Hawaii Good Food Task Force

Chapter Context

Managing and implementing government-regulated programs that make a difference and have meaningful impact was never an easy task. That task became especially difficult while I was a program manager at the Department of Health trying to implement a traditional USDA nutrition education program as the funding platform for a project to increase healthy eating among Supplemental Nutrition Assistance Program (SNAP)-eligible populations. The USDA restrictive structured template approach was diametrically opposed to the public health philosophy of facilitated community-driven strategies and implementation. As a person rooted in public health and community-based approaches, this created enormous conflict and challenges. By trusting in the wisdom of community and the premise that stakeholder input and involvement was central to effective public health programming, however, we overcame the differences by working with leaders to integrate the USDA program into a public health community-driven framework. Unfortunately, over time the

USDA program grew increasingly structured, inflexible, and mired in admin-istrative politics creating barriers and making differences difficult to navigate. Frustration mounted as we also began to recognize that eating behavior and food systems were intertwined complex problems that could not be addressed with rigid singular strategies.

The traditional approaches were not working and seemed inadequate and untenable. The partnerships and synergies we experienced while working with communities led to an epiphany that things could be done differently. We began to look for solutions outside of the program, even as I retired. Determined to build food systems using approaches and strategies that met the needs particular to each community to initiate change, our community leaders embarked on a journey to organize and develop a different construct: a network of community-based food system networks aligned around common goals and a vision to promote food justice and equitable access to good food as avenues to good health and well-being.

The following chapter describes our journey as we evolved into a "network of networks," how we arrived at such framework, the elements that led to our success, as well as the challenges we faced as we established a strong cohesive alliance. The key to our strength and development was listening to commu-nities and following their lead. In addition, we put concerted, conscious effort into establishing and building a culture of trust, loyalty, and collaboration among all members. These critical elements contribute to our continuing commitment and success.

Introduction

From the start, we knew making healthy eating a social norm in Hawaii's low-income communities would be an enormous undertaking. We understood that eating behavior was influenced by a host of social and cultural norms and issues. We hadn't fully comprehended, however, how much it was also affected by the economic, political, and social complexities related to food systems and mechanisms of accessibility, availability, and affordability. As we delved deeper into our work, we quickly learned that all of these issues need to be addressed simultaneously to achieve even small movements toward change. The issues and complexities presented were so overwhelming that identifying where and how to begin posed a challenge.

We decided to simply follow our instincts. Given that our basic tenet was that all project development should be community informed and community driven, we turned to our community leaders to lead the way. They began by designing culturally sensitive programs and strategies that engaged community members to vest and take interest in healthy eating, partnering with multiple organizations and sectors to make existing food hubs and systems more effective and efficient in making produce more accessible and affordable in their communities. We found communities designing and developing unique networks, shaping their community food systems to address the concerns particular to them. Eventually, what ensued was the development of the Hawaii Good Food Alliance, a "network of networks" approach to connect and strengthen food systems across our local communities. Our mission evolved into a strategy of supporting local leaders to transform and establish effective food systems at the grassroots level, then intersecting the leaders and their networks into a united effort to share best practices, provide support to one another, and cross collaborate to generate change at a broader level.

Ultimately, we developed an approach that coincidentally aligned with networking and leadership strategies documented by Meehan and Holley for facilitating social movement. In this chapter, we describe how the Hawaii Good Food Alliance evolved, how we arrived at this strategy, and the lessons learned along the way.

Our Journey toward a Network Strategy

Our story begins around 2007, as obesity emerged as a major public health issue in the United States. The Hawaii Department of Health (DOH) was charged with changing eating behavior and addressing obesity among Supplemental Nutrition Assistance Program (SNAP)-eligible populations through the US Department of Agriculture (USDA) SNAP-Education (Ed) program (formally known as the Food Stamp Nutrition Education—FSNE program). At that time little was known about effective strategies for changing eating behavior, and public health strategies for preventing obesity were uncharted. Increasing fruit and vegetable consumption was indicated as a promising approach. The USDA focused on targeting individuals through one-on-one direct nutrition information delivery while the Centers for Disease Control and Prevention (CDC) Recommended Community Strategies for obesity prevention were yet to be developed.

The Initial Pilot (in Kalihi)

Initially we were searching for any clues that might help us have an impact on a person's eating behavior. Falling back on basic public health principles, the DOH decided to design our own so-called comprehensive integrated multipronged community approach—basically a plan to mass disseminate "eat more fruits and vegetables" messages in communities through multiple channels using a combination of direct education programs through individual community organizations, cross-organization community projects and initiatives, and an overarching social marketing campaign to reinforce the message in hopes this would somehow influence our target population to change eating habits.

We reached out to three community organizations: (1) Kalihi Palama Health Center (Kalihi Palama), (2) Kokua Kalihi Valley Comprehensive Family Services (KKV), and (3) the YMCA, and funded them to implement USDA direct education programs in their organizations. We piloted this approach in the generally low-income community of Kalihi (a three-mile radius area adjacent to downtown Honolulu), which consists of over fifteen different immigrant Pacific Islander ethnic groups, many newly immigrated and difficult to reach. The organizations were also asked to work in committee to collaborate and develop joint community initiatives that would be culturally appropriate and effective in reaching diverse ethnic immigrant populations.

As with any beginning, establishing this group required a great deal of concentrated energy and effort, and constant study and examination of the problems confronting them. The committee met monthly. The first few meetings were somewhat awkward and forced because the organizations had never worked together and didn't know what to expect. Underlying relationships and territories needed to be respected. We constantly worked at building relations between organizations, building trust and loyalty among members, nudging people to attend meetings, finding projects that had common value and benefit to the organizations, carefully planning and executing meeting agendas that were meaningful and did not waste people's time, and even providing food to attract members to attend meetings. Much effort was put into orchestrating gatherings and attending to members' needs and expectations to achieve buy-in. The task was difficult in that this responsibility fell on one person, the SNAP-Ed program manager, because of limited DOH staffing.

Pursuing this path proved valuable, however. Working with community helped us find more effective approaches to effect change. Kalihi Palama engaged small groups using hands-on cooking activities and printed recipe cards with attractive photos of food and step-by-step instructions using pictures and illustrations rather than words. In using this approach, people actually took interest in trying new recipes on their own. We were able to compare this result with similar results observed in a separate project in which elementary school students participated in gardening activities and engaged in cooking potluck dinners for their parents using produce from their harvest. The students not only eagerly ate fruits and vegetables but even asked for them as snacks during the school day. More amazingly, the parents and neighbors living around the school garden soon started to partake in the produce and began protecting the garden from vandalism. We learned from these community strategies that it wasn't messaging but hands-on participatory activities that influenced and moved people to try new foods and engage in changing behavior.

We learned from KKV the value of partnering with the State Department of Human Services (DHS) to provide SNAP Electronic Benefit Transfer (EBT) access at the nearby city and county farmers market. This led to the passage of a resolution by the Honolulu City Council to provide EBT access at more of its farmers market sites. Meanwhile, we also learned the importance of developing adjunct support programs through the YMCA as it developed a comprehensive K–6 nutrition education and hands-on skills curriculum for its after-school program. Their need to train staff led us to contract our community college culinary arts department to develop a six-week train-the-trainer healthy cooking skills program for the YMCA, which was subsequently used to train staff in other community organizations.

Through insisting the three organizations support and participate in each other's activities and programs, camaraderie developed, which resulted in the sharing and expansion of activities across all of the organizations and into the community. They investigated EBT benefit access and Double Up Food Bucks programs for all of the nearby farmers markets, provided cooking skills training in their organizations, while the YMCA organized a Junior Chef competition program that attracted involvement from additional organizations across the community. Their collaboration culminated in a joint twelve-week community-wide social marketing campaign involving radio ad messaging with the organizations working together to provide associated cooking demonstrations and tasting samples, and packaging fresh produce giveaways for large groups of people at local grocery retailer sites located throughout the community.

Looking back at these simplistic interventions, the learning was not only about strategies for addressing individual behavior but also influencing organizations to recognize and appreciate the value of collaboration and mutual support. Collaboration enabled them to freely reach out and ask for help and resources from one another and create interaction that produced amplified impact in the community. Following these events, the group developed a logo and adopted the name Live Better Together Collaborative (LBT Collaborative) to reflect their synergy and the culture and values of their community.

With success in Kalihi, momentum accelerated, and partnership opportunities opened. In keeping with collective impact theory to be inclusive and collaborate collectively, we invited influencers from a multitude of sectors (from DHS, city council representatives, major health insurers, the Parks and Recreation Department, the community college culinary arts department to farmers markets as well as grocery retailers providing venues for activities—even catching the attention of the governor and lieutenant governor's offices). This helped us garner additional resources and attention to better meet the needs of the Kalihi community.

When we thought our work was around one or a few specific issues, such as educating the public to eat healthy, collective impact theory was effective in helping us gather partners to collaborate and generate synergy. When we realized the issue was much more involved and complex, that we needed to address the influences of food supply chains and issues of availability and affordability, we had to formulate an expanded theory of change.

Beginnings of Networks

Fortunately, as we were busily occupied with gathering bits of information regarding strategies for influencing eating behavior, KKV was slowly assembling the elements of a community cultural food hub. As it conducted gardening and cooking programs in nearby schools and public housing projects as directed by DOH funding, it obtained grant funding from the Wholesome Wave organization to add a Double Up Food Bucks program to the EBT benefit access program it initiated at the local city and county farmers market. KKV also built greenhouses and expanded its community garden project to provide produce for its staff and patients, built a café within its community health center, and reached out to community members to develop activities and events that celebrated cultural and indigenous foods.

From an outside view, these activities appeared to be a random set of projects. When KKV was ready and finally linked them all into a cultural food hub, we realized they had created a unique framework for supporting and strengthening healthy culturally informed eating across its community. KKV had implemented its own version of a comprehensive integrated multipronged community approach and had developed a community food systems network by linking and intersecting multiple programs, strategies, partners, and sectors into a dynamic framework. It addressed the cultural uniqueness of their community and demonstrated respect and support for the community's population, resulting in an effective approach for influencing eating norms. KKV continued to expand this hub by organizing a small collective of farmers to increase provision of indigenous produce in Kalihi, integrated youth empowerment and the Junior Chef programs, and established a comprehensive cultural food system that has become the hallmark of an indigenous good food movement in Hawaii.

Springing from the success in Kalihi, we turned to replicating the collaborative model on the Big Island (Hawaii). We contracted the Kohala Center, an independent, community-based center for research, conservation, and education, to establish a LBT Collaborative on the Big Island. While the Big Island community leaders readily collaborated, they had a different strategy in mind for addressing healthy eating. Because the island was large and predominately rural, access to fresh fruits and vegetables in remote areas was its biggest concern. Initially the program emphasis was on assisting farmers markets to accept EBT, a strategy with significant success in food desert areas. The Kohala Center then formed a partnership with the Food Basket, their local food bank, to develop a different food hub. This food hub utilized food bank trucks, empty after delivering canned goods to food pantry sites, to collect fruit and vegetables from farmers to create Community Supported Agriculture (CSA) boxes for distribution back at various food pantry sites located throughout the island. The CSA boxes were sold through EBT benefits or at a discounted price. Nutrition education with cooking demonstrations, hands-on activities, and social marketing were incorporated to encourage their recipients to consume more fruits and vegetables.

About that time, the Blue Zones project was introduced on the Big Island. The Hawaii Department of Health's LBT Collaborative merged with the Blue Zones project to develop the Hawaii Island Food Alliance, linking farmers, the local grocery retailer chain, the government, and representatives from multiple sectors throughout the island to form a food system networking group. The LBT concept had morphed into a different integrated comprehensive community multipronged approach, requiring DOH to modify its original concept of replicating collaborative models statewide under the same title. We were forced to recognize that each community needed autonomy and the ability to network and collaborate in their own way. We learned, in doing so, that the resulting collaboratives were much more effective in reaching community.

With the addition of the Hawaii Island collaborative, the LBT Collaborative was propelled to a new level. In an attempt to nudge Kalihi and the Big Island to share and work across collaboratives and islands, monthly meetings—which had previously been held as gatherings of local Kalihi partners in a room at the YMCA—suddenly expanded to monthly interisland phone conferences of fifteen people. To our surprise, as difficult as it was for a large group of people to meet over the phone, leaders on the Waianae Coast as well as in the Waimanalo and Waianae communities of Oahu, and the island of Molokai, all struggling to help their communities develop healthy food access programs, soon joined in the calls. We had suddenly expanded into a statewide collaborative.

Faced now with a wide array of members, issues, and concerns, a diverse set of communities, and limited resources, the quandary was figuring out how to support all of these community efforts. We thought a solution would be to arm the leaders with community organizing training, providing them with tools with which they could organize to take charge of developing community food hubs and food systems on their own. In attending the training, what the leaders found most valuable was face-to-face networking with others dealing with the same issues. It became apparent what the communities really needed was to be connected in order to share resources and ideas with each other. We realized some person or body needed to coordinate and set up meetings to make this possible.

Transition to a Networking Community Networks Framework

Up to this point, the SNAP-Ed program manager was functioning as a one-person backbone, organizing meetings and deciding the direction and agenda for the LBT Collaborative. As the membership multiplied it was clear the leaders were facing much more complex issues than simply nutrition education. Expertise beyond public health and nutrition education was needed in areas such as sustaining agricultural production, increasing overall food supply, stimulating economic development, obtaining financing, farmer education and training, job development, food banking, and food distribution. Moving toward the idea of facilitating self-sustaining community food systems, the SNAP-Ed manager recruited the leaders of the Big Island collaborative to form a backbone team with broader expertise to guide the work of the expanding statewide collective. The five-member team was called the Hawaii Good Food Task Force.

Given the complex array of issues, values, and beliefs connected to food, the task force took an important pause to examine and define its mission. We decided that carving a narrow niche within which to focus would be more effective and would result in greater impact rather than trying to address a diverse array of issues and concerns among a wide audience of partners. We determined that our purpose was to support leaders in building community-based food system networks to improve access and healthy eating among low-income populations. Our mission was to support and foster these networks and connect them into a larger cohesive initiative to effect social transformation on a larger scale.

The greatest transition for the collaborative occurred at this juncture, when the SNAP-Ed manager retired from DOH, which meant the collaborative would no longer have access to funding or resources from the initial government channel. Because the task force was composed of members who were extremely committed to community well-being and making a difference, they decided to find other avenues of support. In other words, the collaborative was continuing with an unpaid volunteer at the helm with no idea how to fund or continue the initiative.

To complete a contract held by the Kohala Center, the task force assisted Ken Meter (Crossroads Resource Center) to conduct and publish a baseline study on the status of food in low-income communities in Hawaii titled "Hawaii Food for All." In doing so, the task force stayed in touch with the community leaders who had been involved in the LBT Collaborative. When asked if they were interested in continuing as a network group, the collaborative leaders overwhelmingly assented. KKV donated their café as the meeting venue, neighbor island leaders funded their own flights to Honolulu, and attendees paid for their own lunches. And so, the community leaders network reunited under the temporary name of the Hawaii Good Food Network (the Network).

Shortly after this point the Network was able to gain support through the retired SNAP-Ed manager's participation in the Robert Wood Johnson Foundation (RWJF) Culture of Health Leaders Program (CoHL). This provided validation and recognition for the Network and our approach to food systems change. Through the RWJF fellowship and opportunities for the SNAP-Ed manager, KKV, and the Big Island leaders to present the "Hawaii Food for All" study at the New Entry Community Food Systems Conference in Boston in 2017 and again at the Wallace National Good Food Network in Albuquerque in 2018, the Network gained recognition and attention for its "Network of Networks" model. What followed were opportunities for coordination funding.

Re-Structuring the Network of Networks Framework (Hawaii Good Food Alliance)

Fortunately, during this formative period, the task force connected with Islander Institute, a highly regarded facilitation team, to conduct a Network meeting. Looking at the variety and diversity of members into which the Network had grown, the facilitators suggested we reexamine our membership to align with our purpose and goals. It was a difficult process to pare down membership and partners who had started with the collaborative from the beginning. With the guidance of Islander Institute and after a great deal of discussion, the membership was narrowed to community leaders who were developing food distribution systems that connected production to the community and served low-income populations. This was a turning point in the framework of the Network. The membership became more coherent and aligned in purpose and goals and consisted of members focused solely on building food networks in their communities. Former members were asked to allow us time to reconfigure our base and strategies before reexpanding. The facilitators became vested partners in the Network.

The Network managed to continue without dedicated resources, cobbling bits of extra funding to meet. It was fortuitous at this juncture that the Louie Family Foundation, a private family foundation on the mainland, took an interest in our work and provided a small, but critical, sum of gap funding to enable a retreat in January 2018. At that retreat, the Network members bonded, became highly committed, and began working on a charter of agreed values and goals, resulting in a focused and well-articulated purpose statement. The lesson at this juncture was that aligning membership and staying targeted on a specific mission and agreed-upon strategies is an imperative. We ended up with a strongly committed group of twenty-seven leaders from eighteen distinct organizations, representing eight communities throughout the state who were determined to mobilize a good food movement in Hawaii. The group renamed itself the Hawaii Good Food Alliance (Alliance) and chose the word *alliance* to signify their commitment to taking an activist-advocate role rather than being just an information-sharing network. Because of group commitment, the Alliance came out a stronger and more unified organization.

Vision for the Future

As our community-based members continue to expand their work, we envision they will increase and extend their linkages, and intersect with other sectors and networks in Hawaii. As more and more organizations interconnect, we hope to create a culture of health in Hawaii where people value the norm that good food is important and should be affordable and available to everyone in the state, regardless of socioeconomic status.

Through the statewide Alliance communities, we have developed a framework and a platform for improving food systems and support for a social movement toward healthy eating for everyone.

Lessons

What led the Alliance to develop and engage in network strategy was the realization that food and food systems were highly complex and that the issues presented by them could not be solved with conventional linear intervention models. We decided that there were issues and problems so large and complex that it required approaches involving multiple leaders working collectively and collaboratively at multiple foci to meet challenges such as those presented by interconnected, dynamic, complex food systems.

We found our way by listening to and following communities and by allowing for experimentation and learning. We didn't have a name for it—but saw that by networking and collaborating, we were able to work across organizations, geography, and sector barriers. Our network of networks framework allowed us to reach downstream to address community needs, and influence interpersonal relationships and individual change at the grassroots level while effecting change upstream on a larger scale at the state and societal level. Although this framework is still in development and evolving, we have indications that this model has potential to effect significant impact. The following are the lessons learned as we developed this framework.

Lesson 1: Involve Those Who Are Affected

The most effective solutions came from the people on the ground level. Whether identifying issues or developing solutions, it is essential to involve and trust people on the ground and in the community. People who experience the situation understand best what the issues are and what solutions work. Honoring and following community guidance exhibits respect and sensitivity to the situation, which ultimately leads to appropriate solutions and community vesting in the cause. Moreover, these are key elements for establishing trust and engaging people in the collaboration needed to create synergy for social change.

Lesson 2: Community Must Always Be Front and Center

Above all else, the greater community good must be in the front and center as the guiding principle and North Star of the group and its work. All decisions and activities must be dictated by what is good for community. Each member of a collaborative change team must have genuine sincerity and commitment to the work of community over self-interest. Beliefs and values held by individual members eventually permeate and influence every relationship and, ultimately, every aspect of an organization. Thus, it is important all members hold the same core values.

Lesson 3: Maintain High Standards of Values

Maintaining a high standard of values sustains morale and the sense of integrity needed to promote commitment and sustainability. Over time, whether members stay committed, relationships are kept, and the organization/cause is sustained, depends on complete authenticity and sincerity.

Lesson 4: Having a Clear Vision and Purpose Is Vital

Having a consistent clear vision and purpose is key for the existence and sustainability of the group. Without a clear idea of the end goal and purpose of the group, the group will flounder and eventually fall apart.

It also helps maintain trust and respect among members because each person understands their role and the end goal better. Trust in relationships must be continuously nurtured and guarded.

Lesson 5: Have a Coordinator

Whether it's one person or a team, a coordinating entity should exist to keep network members working together, more specifically: organized, coordinated, meeting regularly, communicating with one another, and on track with respect to core values. The backbone must be tenacious and committed to keeping the group together and moving forward. In the initial phases this backbone was critical in setting the culture of the network. The network's backbone organization must also be capable of making difficult decisions while differentiating relationships and issues to protect the startup of the organization.

Our coordinator worked behind the scenes constantly to facilitate and build relationships, check in, and get feedback from members one-on-one. They also ensured misunderstandings were resolved and that concerns were addressed. The coordinator must be forward-looking—constantly watching for opportunities, challenges, and barriers and be willing to confront the group with preparations.

Lesson 6: An Unbiased Facilitator Was Helpful

The facilitator ensures leadership biases do not go unchecked. Furthermore, they offer an outsider's perspective for reflection to reduce chances of misreading of circumstances.

Lesson 7: Leaders Conscientiously Monitor and Align the Vision, Mission, and Goals of the Collaborative

In order to move forward effectively, someone or some steering group must have a clear idea about the group's purpose, what needs to be accomplished, and how to accomplish it. Complex systems constantly change. Therefore, leadership must diligently monitor changes in opportunities, the environment, and the group itself. In our case, we developed a network of networks theory of change. When we observed networks making a difference as they created relationships and partnerships to form local food hubs and food systems that successfully engaged the community, we linked those networks into a larger community of networks.

Lesson 8: Developing a Collaborative Requires Intentional Relationship Building

Building cohesion is not a willy-nilly process. Instead, it is the result of deliberate and thoughtful assessment of members for common goals, values, purpose, and capacity to work collaboratively. Intentionally building relationships and trust further cements clear visions and goals. Carefully vetting members ensured they were aligned with regards to values, mission, commitment level, and working style. This helps foster a group mindset, which leads to a far greater impact.

Lesson 9: Constant, Clear, and Transparent Communication Is Paramount

Constant, clear, and transparent communication among all members is fundamental and essential to building trusting relationships as well as keeping everyone informed and involved. The backbone, or coordinator, needs to communicate with members constantly. Likewise, members should be able to initiate communication with others in the group freely and with transparency.

Lesson 10: Creating Change Is Not Easy

The journey of developing a collaborative is long and arduous, and requires tenacity. The process is not linear, predictable, or controllable. Your group must have foresight, flexibility, stamina, and vision to navigate and sustain the challenges of making change.

Challenges

Networking is an emerging theory of change to address monumental, complex problems where conventional, linear strategies and interventions are ineffective. Networking organizations often take time to develop and often need to change course and adapt to changing dynamic environments. Current conventional funder strategies need to be adjusted to accommodate this different paradigm. Coordination and formation of coordinating infrastructure must be supported to enable networks to survive long enough to begin implementing change strategies.

Burnout is inevitable. Networking takes commitment over a long period of time, often with inadequate or no funding. Sustaining the momentum without support is a challenge and requires grit. Networking is dynamic and requires a different method of accountability and evaluation (developmental evaluation). In our experience, we found networks to be valuable as they enable intersection, cross-pollination of ideas and resources, and cross-organizational collaboration, which can transcend geographical and sector boundaries and mobilize synergy with greater magnitude to create social change. The challenge lies in developing new ways of thinking and funding to accommodate this different paradigm.

References

Harvard Business Review. 2015. *Harvard Business Review's 10 Must Reads: On Emotional Intelligence*. Cambridge, MA: Harvard Business Review Press.

Leadership Learning Community. 2017. *Leading Culture and Systems Change: How to Develop Network Leadership and Support Emerging Networks*. http://leadership learning.org/leading-culture-and-systems-change-how-to-develop-network -leadership-and-support-emerging-networks.

Meehan, D., and C. Reinelt. 2012. *Leadership and Networks: New Ways of Developing Leadership in a Highly Connected World*. http://leadershiplearning.org/leader ship-resources/resources-and-publications/leadership-and-networks-new -ways-developing-leader-0.

Meehan, D., C. Reinelt, and S. Leiderman. 2015. *Leadership and Large-Scale Change*. http://leadershiplearning.org/system/files/2015%20Leadership%20Large%20 Scale%20Change.pdf.

Chapter 5

One Community, Two Voices

Shannon McGuire
Spark Strategic Solutions

Jean Mutchie
St. Luke's Children's Hospital

Chapter Context

Watching my ten-year-old daughter interact with her classmates at a low-resourced school, I (Jean) was struck by hope and possibility. The majority of those children hadn't yet classified their friends by ethnicity, income level, gender, or by where they lived. The children would openly share their dreams, they lifted one another up when they were sad, and they helped when someone was lonely. They saw each other as one community. But, when the doors closed at the end of the day, many of those kids returned to areas of our community where disparities sharply contrasted the experiences they had at school. Many families were struggling to meet basic needs, some parents were incarcerated, help with homework was often minimal, playing outside didn't always feel safe, food could be scarce, and many felt like they held less value in the eyes of our community. Inequity drew a stark line for far too many children where I live.

I believe every child should have the opportunity to fulfill their promise and potential, and that is deeply rooted in the objective of the change I want to see in my community. I believe that the community narrative is imperative to seek to inform and contextualize the benefits and barriers that exist within segments of our community. Data is a critical element, and collaborative voices—led by those seeking change—are fundamental. Moving the needle against inequity is fundamental to creating a culture of health. It must be more than aspirational—the future of our children depends on it.

Community data and voice has been the catalyst to shaping change in specific census tracts within Nampa. The work is rife with complexity, but there seems to be willingness to link arms with intentionality around our children. A community healthy conditions assessment provided data that is irrefutable and offered a pathway for collaboration that had not existed previously. With specific focus around improving access to healthy foods, addressing housing spectrum challenges, improving transportation options, and applying an equity lens to the change process, coalition building became more intentional. The Healthy Impact Nampa Coalition emerged as a result, and having some dedicated funding support through the Blue Cross of Idaho Foundation for Health has allowed projects and initiatives to prove successful. Data is, and will continue to be, a critical element, and collaborative voices, led by those seeking change, are fundamental. Having significant positive impact on inequity is fundamental to creating a culture of health.

As part of a healthcare system my focus is finding solutions that combine population and community health strategies to improve health equity for all residents of my community—with a specific focus on our children. I believe that cross-sector collaboration is imperative to building a culture of health in communities. When residents feel their voice is heard and they have the power to influence change, there is very little that can't be accomplished.

The change process can be complex, however. Resident engagement has been difficult to sustain due to a high mobility rate in the neighborhoods. The lack of a consistent neighborhood champion voice has made the work more challenging at times, but there have been some really impactful changes. A free grocery store shuttle now runs through two of the census tracts most impacted by food deserts. Additionally, a high school has partnered with the neighborhood and community collaborators to begin the Traveling Table—a mobile food pantry that moves to various locations to decrease transportation barriers for those needing access to food.

Since the beginning of the project, our community has had a mayoral change. The new mayor is working with Shannon, this chapter's co-author, to develop a strategic plan to ensure this work is part of the comprehensive plan redesign for the City of Nampa. There is growing understanding and support that linking arms is the most effective way to earn the trust of some of our residents who have felt most marginalized. "Nothing to us, without us" can't be overstated. Let the neighborhood lead the change; sometimes followership is the best leadership.

Introduction

Nampa, Idaho, is nestled among rich agriculture land that drives the economic engine of a growing community. Located twenty miles west of Boise, Nampa is now Idaho's third largest city with a population quickly approaching one hundred thousand residents. A community fundamentally linked by faith and family, stories are regularly shared of those who have called Nampa home for generations.

Although the city has grown, the primary employment sectors have remained relatively consistent: agriculture, railway, manufacturing, and, more recently, significant growth in healthcare. Housing prices have typically been more affordable in Nampa than most areas of the Treasure Valley, so Nampa has long been a commuter community for many seeking to maximize employment opportunities in Boise but returning to a community that was more affordable to live.

Following the Great Recession, however, housing prices began to increase, making home ownership increasingly unattainable for many residents. Additionally, large swaths of land continued to be sold to developers to meet housing demands, but that has also consistently generated concern that the agriculture industry will suffer as land is repurposed.

The community is governed by a mayor and city council, although council members are not elected by district, but rather at-large. This has led to some areas of the community lacking representation by someone who lives in their neighborhood and understands the context of barriers and benefits. Nampa, like the rest of Idaho, is very conservative, and the majority of residents are Republican. This extends to city governance and oversight that largely embraces the free market, very limited government, and very conservative principles. Additionally, tax money is rarely directed toward anything that might be viewed as social equity because it is typically viewed as entitlement spending. Although political ideology may impact the way tax dollars are appropriated, private sector partnerships have shown a willingness to invest in initiatives that improve opportunities for Nampa neighbors.

Having lived in the community for nearly twenty years, Jean Mutchie has had the privilege of linking arms often with community members and businesses invested in making Nampa a great place to live and raise a family. There have been many initiatives started with great intention, but due to lack of funding or sustainability, they have typically stuttered or failed to create the anticipated impact.

Data indicated that as Nampa grew, the population of children nineteen years old and younger accounted for more than 35 percent of Nampa's total population (Census 2010). Additionally, a 2010 study conducted by the Idaho Department of Health and Welfare also showed that 30 percent of Idaho third graders were overweight or obese, and Nampa's rate was higher than cities in neighboring Ada County (Forbing-Orr 2012).

That began to change in 2013 when Nampa was awarded a $300,000 High Five Community Transformation Grant through the Blue Cross of Idaho Foundation for Health. The grant was awarded to specifically address an increasing trend in childhood obesity by focusing on increasing access to healthy, affordable food and increasing physical activity.

The grant process included technical assistance that focused on catalyzing engagement and building partnerships to create sustainable change in the community. The grant used data to inform and drive decisions through collaboration among city staff, businesses, organizations, and residents. Additionally, the grant process finally provided the community with a structure for fulfillment that would hopefully lead to sustainability. The grant committee included cross-sector partners from the City of Nampa, the Nampa School District, Nampa Chamber of Commerce, two health systems, public health agencies, community residents, and additional stakeholders interested in decreasing childhood obesity rates in our community.

As the grant work began in earnest, municipal elections were also being held. The incumbent mayor had been very invested in the grant proposal, but he lost to his challenger. Following the election, the new administration was focused on their team's transition, so grant work continued within subcommittees.

One of the subcommittees formed out of the grant process was the Nampa Healthy Kids Coalition. This group began to meet to discuss best practice, multisector approaches to bending the trend of childhood obesity. The group, again, was representative of healthcare, public health, nonprofit agencies, school district personnel, the chamber of commerce, municipal leaders, and city employees. It quickly became apparent to those who had not specifically worked in public health or healthcare that childhood obesity was multifactorial and often very complex.

As the group identified priority areas where funding could have the most impact, much discussion centered on Idaho's determination to forgo expanding Medicaid. There was also continued dialogue about the social determinants of health that were disproportionately influencing poor health for a segment of students in some of our schools. Fortunately, many of us had a great working relationship with Dr. Lindsey Turner, the director of Boise State University's Initiative for Healthy Schools. Dr. Turner's research and work centered on policy, systems, and environmental (PSE) approaches to create sustainable change. Dr. Turner was willing to serve as a coalition member to support the desired change and impact in Nampa.

There had been a discussion about using a large portion of the High Five Community Transformation Grant funds to install new outdoor physical activity equipment at our local recreation facility. The intention was to provide youth with a dedicated space to exercise. As the conversations around policy, systems, and environmental (PSE) change and social determinants of health began to gain momentum, however, the group decided to take a very intentional pause. A very frank and honest conversation was had about the intent of the funding to be catalytic and transformational, neither of which would be achieved by installing very limited fitness equipment in an outdoor gym.

Group dynamics can certainly impact progress, and this decision created disagreement. The new mayor had begun to attend a few meetings of the core grant planning team. He agreed that we needed to think more globally and bigger than fitness equipment, so we began discussing the need to understand our community much better. As easy as this may sound, Nampa was becoming a much more diverse community, and a number of our schools had become majority-minority. Hispanic and Latino residents were beginning to call Nampa home, but many were not realizing the same opportunity to thrive in an improving economy.

At the same time this renewed dialogue was taking place, Nampa had also been selected as one of fifty cities across the United States to receive a Robert Wood Johnson Foundation Invest Health grant. The ability to have both grants work in tandem created exciting synergy. Shannon McGuire, chief empowerment officer of Spark!, had begun consulting with the Blue Cross of Idaho Foundation for Health to manage the High Five Community Transformation grant. Shannon brought an intentional and organic facilitation process that engendered cooperation and collaboration. Under her guidance, previously divergent ideas were forgotten, and the group began to focus intently on maximizing both grant opportunities.

When McGuire began working with the Nampa community, there was tension, mistrust, and confusion among community leaders working on the grant. The challenges stemmed from the conversations around the proposal to install an outdoor gym using grant funds. This was compounded by the election of a new mayor who inherited an initiative that he didn't quite understand. Convinced of the need to support youth, the mayor allocated two-thirds of the grant to invest in school-based initiatives led by the Nampa Healthy Kids Coalition.

Before the group could move forward, a series of conversations were had with each committee member and the group at large to step back and reprioritize intentions, values, and goals of the grant. McGuire led conversations with a focus on learning more about the perceptions and challenges of the collaborative. The individual interviews were eye-opening and revealed where the tensions resided. A few of the key questions asked were:

- Why did you join this collaborative?
- What hopes do you have for youth in Nampa?
- What have been the biggest challenges and frustrations in working together?
- What have been the successes and accomplishments?
- What do you feel the group needs to move forward together?
- Who might be missing from this discussion?

Through the group discussions, the outcomes and issues found in the evaluation were addressed. These weren't easy conversations to have, but the group stuck together and made a commitment to work on resolving the challenges. After spending time on rebuilding group cohesion, the conversation shifted back to what was necessary to make a lasting impact for Nampa's youth.

Information and Data Gathering

Data was foundational to create a feasible plan to generate significant, sustainable change. With McGuire and Dr. Turner as part of the discussion, the grant used a portion of the funding to hire a consultant to conduct an assessment of the health conditions of the City of Nampa. Included in the assessment would be resident surveys and interviews, community leader interviews, content expertise contributions, and census tract-level data around the social determinants of health.

The process for the Nampa Healthy Conditions Assessment would take six months to complete. Throughout the process, and in tandem with the Invest Health grant team, ground-level data was being gathered and other tools were being used to determine the census tracts in Nampa that were being disproportionately impacted by inequities. The data confirmed that two census tracts scored poorly when weighted for the following indicators: poverty, high school graduation rates, homeownership versus renting, greater than 30 percent of income being spent on housing, uninsured rate, percent of Hispanic or Latino residents, qualification for Supplemental Nutrition Assistance Program (SNAP) with children under the age of eighteen, having access to a working vehicle, and the percentage of those living with a disability.

The indicators showed that census tracts 201 and 202 flagged as having the most significant areas of concern. Compounding the challenges faced by residents living in census tract 202, the area had become a food desert due to the two grocery stores closest to the neighborhood permanently closing and limited access to healthy food options. Additionally, parts of census tract 202 had also been designated as a floodway or floodplain by the Federal Emergency Management Agency (FEMA). This designation can make it very expensive for property owners to improve existing structures that will adequately meet the requirements, and the area has become disinvested. The City of Nampa has been disputing the designation with FEMA for years, but it has not yet been resolved (Butts 2008).

The census tract-level data also confirmed that disparities were also evident in health outcomes for residents (Danley 2017). Reported data indicated the following for census tract 202:

- 24.7 percent of adults reported only fair or poor health status (second worst tract in Treasure Valley, second only to downtown Nampa)
- 41.6 percent of adults were reported to be obese, compared to 34 percent for Nampa (the highest rate in Treasure Valley)
- 13.4 percent of adults had been diagnosed with diabetes (tied for the highest rate in Treasure Valley)
- 11.3 percent of adults have asthma (the highest rate in Treasure Valley)
- 30.4 percent of adults were uninsured

This data, along with the data looking at the social determinants of health, painted a rather bleak picture. Census tract 202 had the highest rates of deep generational poverty, low education attainment, lack of access to healthy food, a high number of minority residents, a large number of children living in the neighborhood, and the lowest per capita income in Treasure Valley. It became clear that addressing childhood obesity needed to be done from a causality perspective, and through an equity lens.

Many interviews with residents indicated skepticism and a hesitancy to engage. Neighborhood meetings were held to encourage engagement, and a resident community liaison was hired to help facilitate improved discussion. Residents reported that they often felt their voices were neither heard, nor did they feel they mattered. There was a deep sentiment that they were viewed as the people living on the wrong side of the tracks, and they felt that community leaders didn't respond to their needs.

It was critical to begin creating some momentum for residents to believe that change was possible and that they could lead the effort. The top priorities from the neighborhood survey were identified by resident feedback and prioritized as: (1) access to a grocery store, (2) transportation and connectivity, (3) improved housing quality and better access to affordable housing, and (4) improved access to education and jobs that pay a living wage. Seemingly there should have been some easy momentum in a couple of the priority areas but, as often is the case, some challenges arose.

When the Nampa Healthy Conditions Assessment was completed the data was shared with the mayor and some of his senior administration. There was some initial anger and resistance to the data, along with skepticism of its accuracy and concern about how it would be viewed by the community and other leaders. Following a number of conversations, the mayor determined it needed to be addressed. He was supportive of creating the Healthy Impact Nampa Coalition, a cross-sector group of community leaders focused on addressing the priority areas. The coalition members represent a broad spectrum of community organizations and agencies, but most importantly, residents of north Nampa. The mayor specifically asked only those willing to drive toward action to participate as members of the coalition.

The coalition began working with other groups addressing similar disparities so we could minimize duplication and disparate efforts. Four subcommittees were formed to specifically address food access, the housing spectrum, transportation and connectivity, and early childhood education opportunities. There was a shared understanding that equity was fundamental to creating an opportunity for every resident to have the opportunity to be their healthiest.

Results

The Food Access Committee was able to gain some traction very quickly. It was evident that there was a shortage of food pantries in north Nampa because many households didn't have access to a vehicle. The Idaho Foodbank was a very willing and organized partner, and they determined the data was sufficient to warrant adding a mobile pantry once per month. Having an established coalition and faith organization's support, the mobile pantry became operational very quickly. The pantry continues to provide food to families in north Nampa on the first Wednesday of the month, and one hundred boxes are distributed in less than one hour. There is considerable need yet to be met, but it did create some momentum toward providing some additional food access.

Additionally, the two health systems in Nampa, St. Luke's and Saint Alphonsus, partnered to fund a grocery store shuttle pilot program that runs each Saturday to provide access to a major grocery store. Riders indicated they needed to have prescriptions filled, so the route was changed to include additional access to a store with a pharmacy. The shuttle has been operational for about eight months, and ridership remains very consistent. We are currently working on a sustainability plan with the hospitals, but the city council denied any funding support because they felt it needed to be funded through private sector dollars.

To meet additional food access needs the Traveling Table Mobile Food Pantry became operational in late 2018. The Traveling Table is operated as a partnership between a local leadership high school and a community coalition. The ability to expand access was made possible through the donation of a box truck and a commitment from the Idaho Foodbank to consistently provide food. Fresh produce is being procured locally through faith-based community gardens and individual growers to augment. Using data to inform, the truck operates a set route one day per month to reach our community residents with the highest level of food insecurity. More than three thousand individuals benefited the first year of operations, and there is a need to expand the route in the coming months. Additionally, a dietitian is available to offer recipes and preparation tips to assist in preparing and storing perishable and non-shelf-stable food.

Although these initiatives have increased access to food for many in the neighborhood, there is still a long-term need to reestablish a small neighborhood market again in north Nampa. There is some stated interest in making a market a reality, and we hope to have that materialize over the next two years.

As stated earlier, the political will needed to provide funding has been an ongoing challenge. There has been some movement to address some current zoning policies that might provide improved access to make ancillary dwellings rentable units. The coalition is also addressing opportunities to continue to work with council members to explore the addition of mixed-income properties as well as possible mitigation efforts with FEMA in the hopes of decreasing the expansive area designated as a floodway and flood plain.

We have also faced some similar challenges relative to transportation options for residents. There are limited public transportation options due to little-designated support funding by the City of Nampa. This will likely be one of the more significant challenges faced, so there is much work being led by north Nampa residents with support from the coalition to improve pedestrian and bike-friendly policies and funding. As the community continues to grow, doing nothing will no longer be a viable option. There continues to be committed voices championing policy and system-level change.

As a predominately conservative community, equity has been a topic that continues to require a very intentional conversation to create shared understanding. There seems to be wide agreement that every child should have the opportunity to fulfill their promise and potential. The sobering fact that Nampa has the highest number of children experiencing homelessness in Idaho is not a statistic readily embraced. Under the McKinney-Vento Act, as many as 10 percent of the Nampa student population are qualified as homeless and able to receive assistance. This has created an area to potentially gain traction around the need to address affordable housing, jobs with a living wage, early access to education, and support systems to help every child thrive.

The work is only beginning. Nampa has since had another mayoral change, as well as a new superintendent of the school district. Both women are fully invested in creating a community with unlimited potential. They understand the value of partnerships and collaboration, and they lead and inspire change. The High Five Community Transformation Grant has been a catalyst for conversation, collaboration, and change. The synergy created by the grant created systems thinking change, the determination to take a look at hard truths, change the conversations taking place, challenge assumptions, and engage residents so they lead their own change.

The city motto is "Nampa Proud," and the hope is that it will be true for every resident. This transformational work is foundational to creating a culture of health where every person has a fair and just opportunity to live their healthiest life regardless of race, creed, socioeconomic status, education level, gender identity, or where they live. As a community we have to decide what we value—when one person is lifted, we are all lifted.

Lessons Learned

The story of Nampa's transformation has not been an easy one, but it has been extremely worthwhile. Systems change takes time and investment from those who are committed. Throughout the process of facilitating the change, a few key lessons emerged that may be useful to others on this path. Sometimes there are many barriers to progress that must be addressed.

Lesson 1: Make Sure the Right People Are on the Team

When the High Five Community Transformation Grant began, there were several players involved. As the grant progressed and tensions rose, it was then that the group recognized the voices missing from the conversation. Ensuring that cross-sector collaboration is occurring is a primary focus, but this must also be in connection with engaging the voices of those that will be impacted by the work. In Nampa's case, it was making sure that youth, and youth providers, had a seat at the table.

Lesson 2: Be Willing to Have Hard Conversations

Once tensions rose in relation to the outdoor gym and the results of the Health Conditions Assessment, the initial response was to tiptoe around the conversation. Having an experienced facilitator was extremely beneficial for group progress because it allowed partners the opportunity to voice their concerns, opinions, and desires for change. Throughout the process of the grant, it was clear that conflict had to be managed quickly and efficiently. From the conflict came solutions that led the way to more sustainable solutions for the community.

Lesson 3: Engage Leaders and Influencers from the Start

One of the most significant changes cited throughout Nampa's transformation was the level of leadership engagement and awareness. The mayoral changes that occurred during the beginning of the High Five Community Transformation Grant posed challenges and opportunities. With a new mayor in office, it created a sense of urgency and expectation to get them up to speed on what the grant aimed to do and what partners were working together. In addition to the mayor, involving local leaders in the conversation proved extremely beneficial. Giving them a reason to be involved was key, and the partners shared their enthusiasm and expertise to bring leaders along.

Lesson 4: Communicate, Communicate, and Communicate Some More

One of the major lessons from Nampa's story was the need to have continuous and strategic communication to (and between) partners. This was beyond holding monthly meetings and sending a few emails. It entailed actively listening to each member, engaging in empathetic dialogue, and creating a platform for idea exchange. Having a central source of communication through a designated party helped this process. One source consolidating and sending major communication between the groups also helped ease engagement.

Lesson 5: Use Data to Create Clear Priorities

The action planning process for the High Five Community Transformation Grant began early in the grant process. Setting priorities before there was concrete data created a weak foundation to build on. Once the partnership took a deeper dive into the landscape of the community to better understand the challenges, assets, partnerships, and need, they were able to make more informed decisions. This created greater clarity and a sense of cohesion from which to operate. Using data such as a needs assessment, health conditions assessment, focus groups, community conversations, partner interview, asset mapping, landscape analysis, or systems mapping offers a good starting point for the conversation of funding priorities.

Lesson 6: Give the Funder a Seat at the Table

There are often mixed reviews about including funders at the planning level. In Nampa's case, this was highly beneficial, because it allowed for honest dialogue, two-way communication, a better understanding of expectations from the grantor and grantee, and another set of expertise to provide insight. Having the funder involved in such deep and insightful conversations fostered learning on both ends. Nampa was able to better align its funding priorities to meet specifications and expectations of the foundation by having them involved.

Lesson 7: Leverage Collaboration and Partnerships

Having a core team working together to implement the grant was a true catalyst for the successes in Nampa. By combining resources, knowledge, and focus, the city was able to create many new and unique partnerships that collaborated beyond the initial grant. By forming a network focused on the development of deep and meaningful connection, Nampa was able to begin the shift towards sustainable change. Holding reoccurring meetings and encouraging conversations was key.

Lesson 8: Activate the Champions

Nampa had many champions that were eager and willing to voice their support for the work happening in the community. Finding and engaging these voices helped bridge the gap between practitioners and residents. The partners purposefully sought out individuals that had passion, drive, and credibility to bring awareness to the issues at hand.

References

Butts, M. 2008. "Nampa to Appeal FEMA Flood Map." *Idaho Press*, March 3, 2008. https://www.idahopress.com/news/nampa-to-appeal-fema-flood-map/article _20eb9061–5176-57e3-b04d-be96a967a5a2.html.

Census 2010: Idaho, Nampa. n.d. http://data.spokesman.com/census/2010/idaho/ cities/nampa-id/.

Danley, C. 2017. "Nampa Healthy Conditions Assessment." http://id-nampa.civic plus.com/1163/Data-and-Studies.

Forbing-Orr, N. 2012. "Most Idaho Third Graders Are at a Healthy Weight, but the Percentage of Overweight or Obese Kids is Increasing." Idaho Department of Health and Welfare, December 11, 2012. https://healthandwelfare.idaho.gov/ AboutUs/Newsroom/tabid/130/ctl/ArticleView/mid/3061/articleId/1692/ Most-Idaho-third-graders-are-at-a-healthy-weight-but-the-percentage-of-over weight-or-obese-kids-is-increasing.aspx.

Chapter 6

EMBRacing Community-Engaged Research

Engaging, Managing, and Bonding through Race Intervention

Monique C. McKenny
University of Miami

Riana E. Anderson
University of Michigan

Chapter Context

Monique McKenny's upbringing was full of familial messaging on race and culture. Through this messaging she started to learn about the meaning and implications of race in the lives of black families. As an undergraduate, Monique learned more about research illustrating the pernicious impact of racial discrimination on black youth's development across various domains of functioning. The more literature she read, the more McKenny became overwhelmed with the constant suggestion that black communities were lacking or comparative studies that positioned white families as the norm or standard.

Hundreds of miles away, Dr. Riana Anderson was a then graduate student who was similarly overburdened with deficit language used to describe black families. There is a dearth of literature on the negative impact of discrimination as well as potential protective factors; however, there were no applied interventions to promote health coping among those who experience discrimination. Understanding that a historically oppressive society was the problem and not black families, Anderson sought to develop an intervention that utilized culturally relevant tools to promote racial coping in the face of racial stress resulting from discrimination. Anderson and McKenny ultimately came together to pursue this goal in 2015 at the Racial Empowerment Collaborative in Philadelphia, Anderson as the intervention's developer and McKenny as program coordinator.

While there is a large body of literature documenting the negative impact of discrimination and racial stress, there was no clinical intervention dedicated to the reduction of racial stress and enhancement of racial coping. Further, our intervention, Engaging, Managing, and Bonding through Race (EMBRace) was developed in 2015 by Drs. Riana Anderson and Howard Stevenson to address this need. The intervention seeks to reduce racial stress by bolstering youth and their caregiver's racial self-efficacy, defined as one's perceived ability to effectively resolve racial experiences. Second, the program promotes racial coping by teaching participants healthy coping mechanisms that can be used in response to a racialized event. After participating in EMBRace, it is expected that youth and their caregiver can engage in conversations on race, manage the stress that comes from racialized experiences, and bond with one another in the process.

Together, McKenny and Anderson implemented the intervention with a team of research assistants, clinicians, and developers. After three iterations of the program, they were able to serve over twenty families and develop relationships with several community partners throughout the city. They trained a team of over twenty-five clinicians and research assistants on therapeutic practices to discuss racial stress and racial socialization practices among black families and secured grant funding to sustain the program. They consider this work to have been a success based on the feedback that they received from our clinicians and families, along with preliminary data that illustrates an increase in racial self-efficacy among families who completed the program (Anderson,

McKenny, Koku, Mitchell, and Stevenson 2018). Further, they were able to contribute to the development of racial coping practices for our participating families as well as foster much needed training for a group of clinicians who are now more knowledgeable on how to support youth and families who face racialized stressors.

Throughout the process of developing and implementing the intervention, they as a team learned many lessons, many of which we outline in this chapter. What remains most salient and proved to be vital to our success was being responsive to the feedback given to us by community members and participants. Honoring their needs and embracing participant feedback has been and remains central to the implementation of EMBRace.

Introduction

> *"I got power, poison, pain, and joy inside my DNA."*
>
> —*Kendrick Lamar, "DNA"*

As eloquently intimated by Kendrick Lamar, although black Americans have experienced challenges as a collective, they have also shown great resilience in the face of this struggle through cultural wherewithal. Racial discrimination, for example, continues to be a major social determinant of health on the individual (Carter 2007; Harrell 2000; Williams and Mohammed 2009), community (Brody et al. 2014; Chae et al. 2015), and institutional level (Burgess, Ding, Hargreaves, Van Ryn, and Phelan 2008). Black Americans' experience of racial discrimination has an even greater impact on psychological and physiological health than for European or Latinx Americans (NPR, RWJF, and Harvard University 2017). Over 90 percent of black youth, as young as eight years old, have reported experiencing discrimination within a year's time (Pachter, Bernstein, Szalacha, and Garcia Coll 2010). Youth who report experiencing discrimination

have indicated more depressive symptoms and poorer academic achievement (Neblett, Chavous, Nguyen, and Sellers 2009; Seaton, Caldwell,
Sellers, and Jackson 2010). Similarly, black adults are psychologically
and physiologically impacted by experiences with discrimination, and
reports of discrimination have been linked to cardiovascular disease, poor
sleep, depression, alcohol use, and anxiety (Brown et al. 2000; Metzger et
al. 2018; Slopen, Lewis, and Williams 2016; Williams, Neighbors, and
Jackson 2003). These pernicious effects influence black families as well,
given that parental experiences with discrimination have been linked to
poor parent-child relationships, strained familial bonds, and psychological challenges with children (Anderson et al. 2015).

Despite these challenges, black families have utilized racial socialization, defined as the transaction of verbal and nonverbal messages about
race between caregivers and children, as a tool to equip youth for the
racialized world that they will encounter (Lesane-Brown 2006). Racial
socialization has been studied for decades as a key cultural strength
amongst families of color that has buffered against the deleterious
outcomes related to discrimination. More specifically, racial socialization serves as a protective factor for self-esteem (Harris-Britt, Valrie,
Kurtz-Costes, and Rowley 2007), academic outcomes (Neblett, Philip,
Cogburn, and Sellers 2006), and psychological well-being (Hughes,
Witherspoon, Rivas-Drake, and West-Bey 2009) in the face of discrimination. In a seminal paper, Hughes et al. (2006) identified four tenets
of racial socialization messages that families most often use with their
children. These, ordered by frequency of use, include (1) cultural socialization, (2) preparation for bias, (3) promotion of distrust, and (4) egalitarianism. Cultural socialization refers to messages of racial pride and
those that emphasize the uniqueness of one's racial group. This tenet is
reflected in commonly used phrases like *black is beautiful* or in nonverbal

messages like decorating one's home with black art. Preparation for bias encompasses messages that seek to prepare or equip youth for prejudice or discrimination that they will experience in the world. Examples can be seen when parents explicitly tell children where to put their hands on the wheel if pulled over by police (e.g., "the talk") or how to remove their hood when walking into convenience stores. Promotion of distrust refers to messages of warning against groups of people often based on negative experiences with that group in the past (e.g., "those white people will call the police on you"). Finally, egalitarianism is defined as messages that emphasize the commonalities between all people, suggest we are all one human race, or convey no messages at all about race. Common messages that reflect egalitarian values might include "we're all one human race!" or "race doesn't matter anymore, it's really about how hard you work."

These tenets of racial socialization, particularly the messaging received from parents, have been linked to numerous positive psychosocial outcomes for youth, including academic achievement (Wang and Hughley 2012), psychological well-being (Neblett, Smalls, Ford, Nguyen, and Sellers 2009), adolescent coping (Anderson, Jones, Anwiyo, McKenny, and Gaylord-Harden 2018), and self-efficacy (Bowman and Howard 1985). The Racial Encounter, Coping, Appraisal, and Socialization Theory (RECAST), furthermore, posits that racial socialization is a dynamic process of transactions between parent and child based on building self-efficacy through intentional practice and the development of competence (Anderson and Stevenson 2019). Through racial socialization, youth and families can begin to read and recast their racial experiences to begin healing together.

Given the protective value of racial socialization in psychosocial outcomes for youth, scholars have called for the continued integration of racial socialization into family-and community-based interventions

(Jones and Neblett 2018). Interventions utilizing racial socialization have been effective in promoting self-esteem (Sisters of Nia; Belgrave, Reed, Plybon, and Corneille 2004; Black Parenting Strengths and Strategies [BPSS]; Coard, Foy-Watson, Zimmer, and Wallace 2007), discouraging drug use (Strong African American Families Program; Brody, Yi-Fu, Kogan, Murry, and Brown 2010), and managing aggression (Preventing Long-Term Anger and Aggression in Youth [PLAAY]; Stevenson 2003). Coard et al. (2007) engaged groups of black parents in discussions around their parenting strengths and challenges, while Stevenson (2003) integrated the theoretical components of RECAST in the PLAAY intervention to help young boys process racial incidents and their resulting anger through physical play on the basketball court. Despite the abundance of literature emphasizing the deleterious impact of discrimination on the health of black youth and families (Williams et al. 2003) and the buffering role of racial socialization, no interventions had been specifically developed for these race-related phenomena in black families.

Based on the theoretical implications of RECAST (Anderson and Stevenson 2019) and building on existing interventions that utilized racial socialization to promote positive health outcomes for black youth (PLAAY) and parents (BPSS), a new intervention was conceptualized, developed, and implemented. Engaging, Managing, and Bonding through Race (EMBRace; Anderson and Stevenson 2016) sought to support African American families in effectively *engaging* in racial messages, *managing* racial stress and trauma from racial encounters, and *bonding* with their children in the process. Within this chapter, EMBRace developer Dr. Riana Anderson, now an assistant professor at the University of Michigan's School of Public Health, and former EMBRace program coordinator Monique McKenny, now a doctoral student at the University of Miami's School of Education and Human Development, will discuss the process of developing and implementing this intervention in Philadelphia. Pivotal and enlightening experiences from implementation will be shared in light of the personal histories of the staff. Finally, we offer personal reflections and calls for action in community collaboration and activism to address health disparities related to social determinants of health, like racial discrimination, in novel and effective ways.

What is EMBRace?

EMBRace was developed from decades of research showing how racial encounters impact the health and well-being of black adults, youth, and families and the theoretical premises of RECAST. RECAST suggests that just as an individual can learn to read and develop literacy for text, individuals can learn, practice, and develop literacy for understanding and addressing racial encounters. For youth and families, this literacy is developed through racial socialization. As such, EMBRace is a seven-week family-level intervention that focuses on engaging parents in conversations on race, thus enriching racial socialization literacy. While much of the literature on racial socialization focuses on the frequency of racial socialization messaging, EMBRace is interested in the competency or efficacy that parents develop in discussing difficult racial matters with their children, and similarly, how efficacious youth feel in discussing racial matters with their caregivers. Second, EMBRace seeks to help families manage racial stress and trauma. Racial stress and trauma resulting from racial discrimination may account for a number of health disparities among black communities (Williams et al. 2003). EMBRace incorporates coping strategies specifically developed to target racialized stress for black families (Stevenson 2003). Among the strategies utilized in the intervention are storytelling, journaling, "comeback lines," and calculate, locate, communicate, breathe, and exhale (CLC-BE). CLC-BE is a mindfulness practice in which the individual calculates, locates, and communicates his or her stress, then breathes and exhales. Finally, through principals of affection, correction, and protection, families are encouraged to bond with one another and improve the parent-child relationship.

The first and last weeks of EMBRace consist of a variety of assessments—for example, surveys, interviews, and observations—that provide a holistic representation of participant well-being. Within the middle five weeks of the intervention, parents and children complete various tasks, including a family tree, role playing, and storytelling to work through each of the four tenets of racial socialization. The sessions are co-led by the participating family and their clinicians, two people with whom they work consistently over the course of the program. EMBRace is a family-level intervention, not a group intervention, so parents get to work exclusively with their children and clinicians each week.

A typical EMBRace session is ninety minutes long and is divided into three parts. Within the first thirty minutes of the session, the parent and child separate to discuss the tenet of the week—for example, cultural socialization; week one—and their experiences related to this tenet. This time apart from one another allows the parent and child to process racial encounters individually with their clinician. To illustrate the importance of this approach, if a parent is talking to their child about a recent murder publicized by the media, the parent not only has to engage with the youth but also has to manage their own trauma about the racial incidents they have experienced or imagine their children experiencing. While the literature indicates that racial socialization is often utilized to protect the youth from racist experiences, very few applied methods have explored the ways parents can protect their internalized pain throughout the process.

Families then break to share a meal for fifteen minutes. This meal also serves as an opportunity for rapport building between clinicians and the family while underscoring the communal nature of the intervention. The final forty-five minutes of the session calls for the parent and child to reunite in the presence of both of their clinicians, to complete tasks together—for example, family tree; week one—receive psychoeducation ("research has shown that youth who receive self-worth messages from their parents have more positive academic outcomes. These messages may counteract the negative impact of discrimination"; Neblett, Philip, Cogburn, and Sellers 2006), and have a discussion on the tenet of the week—for example, "do you think it is important to be proud of your race?"). For further discussion of the structure and components of the intervention, see Anderson, McKenny, and Stevenson (2018).

Research Process

Following the scientific method used in various disciplines, the development and implementation of EMBRace began with an observation. Drs. Riana Anderson and Howard Stevenson identified the need for a culturally relevant intervention for black youth and families who face racial encounters. Despite the abundance of literature illuminating the impact of racial stress on black youth, there was no intervention focused specifically on racial coping for these young people and their families. Intervention development began with a literature review of empirical research and existing interventions for this population. Among these interventions (e.g., PLAAY, BPSS, SAAF, Sisters of Nia), cultural relevance and the utilization of existing cultural strengths (e.g., racial socialization) of the population were identified as important aspects of the interventions' efficacy.

After seven months of literature reviews, meetings, and drafting, the EMBRace manualized curriculum was prepared to incorporate: (1) psychoeducation from the racial socialization literature, (2) culturally relevant racial coping strategies, and (3) opportunities for parent-child communication to be strengthened. The development of the manual drew on researchers and clinicians from various disciplines, including clinical psychology, counseling psychology, social work, and education. Similarly, the implementation of the intervention would require expertise in various interpersonal areas as we sought to take the intervention from the lab to the community. A manual was finalized consisting of pre-and post-tests and five content sessions. After development, community partners were established, and collaborative planning allowed for developers, community partners, and clinicians to identify a start date.

Our next task was to assemble and train a team of individuals to administer the intervention. Simultaneously, we sought to find community partners and a home for the intervention at a local school in a predominantly black West Philadelphia community. Training occurred prior to intervention start dates. Intervention staff (clinicians and research assistants) and community partner staff (e.g., teachers, school social workers, etc.) were introduced prior to intervention start dates.

The first iteration ran throughout the spring semester of an academic year. At the close of the first iteration, principal investigators utilized the summer to assess the intervention progress, acceptability, and feasibility of EMBRace (see Anderson, McKenny, Mitchell, Koku, and Stevenson 2017). Focus groups were held with youth and parents from the community for feedback. A program coordinator was hired for the forthcoming iteration through the receipt of grant funding. The intervention manual was revised for clinician ease and clarity. Protocols were strengthened as the intervention prepared to serve more families in the second iteration.

In this section, we will discuss the process of implementing the intervention during the first and second phase of piloting. We conclude by highlighting lessons learned between these two iterations.

Staff and Training

The EMBRace staff consisted of several roles, including developers, program coordinators, clinicians, and research assistants. Clinicians and research assistants for the first iteration of EMBRace were recruited from the Racial Empowerment Collaborative, a laboratory led by Dr. Howard Stevenson, the co-developer of EMBRace. Many members from the development team volunteered to serve as clinicians in the intervention. These volunteers ranged from masters' students to postdoctoral fellows in the Graduate School of Education. For many of the masters' level volunteers, their participation in EMBRace drew from their counseling training, including tools necessary for the implementation of therapeutic intervention. In later iterations, clinicians were recruited from local universities with training programs in psychology and marriage and family therapy. Research assistants were also recruited in a similar fashion. The research assistant position was ideal for students who wanted to gain research experience but did not have the desire or training to dedicate to clinical work and supervision.

The training of intervention staff was led by the intervention developers. Research assistants and clinicians attended one conjoined training session to build rapport within the team and to address overarching topics that would be central to everyone's work in EMBRace. Within this first overarching training session, team members were encouraged to consider their social positioning and biases. We believed it was imperative that team members examined themselves before working with parents and youth on sensitive topics of race, bias, and prejudice to avoid the transference of microaggressions or trauma. Additionally, in order for clinicians to create a safe, therapeutic space in which participants could recall racial traumas and learn racial coping, team members needed to sit with their own social positions and privileges. Following our initial training, research assistants and clinicians were trained separately on their specific roles.

Throughout EMBRace, we have been a team composed of individuals from various racial and ethnic backgrounds. Our team has consistently been predominantly people of color including research assistants and clinicians who identified as black, Asian, and Latinx. Although we initially hesitated to include white clinicians and research assistants, we understood that they maintain the largest percentage of students and trainees within this field and knew it was equally, if not more, important to train them to be culturally competent. Furthermore, our white clinicians, along with our clinicians of color, both illuminate a larger goal of the developers in better educating practitioners and researchers from various racial backgrounds on the culturally specific needs of populations of color. At the conclusion of EMBRace, participants were asked if racial differences between their clinician and their family impacted their experience in the program. While some families did express feeling the need to "filter" their words based on the clinician's racial background, others explained that their clinician's racial background did not matter to them once solid rapport was built.

Lessons Learned

(1) Incorporate sociocultural training for intervention staff that continues throughout their tenure in the program. (2) Request feedback from

participants throughout the intervention and have clinicians explicitly discuss how race and racial differences can impact the space.

Partnerships

In an effort to recruit youth and families as well as identify a convenient space within the participants' communities, EMBRace has sought partnerships with schools and other youth-serving organizations. Relying on established connections strengthened by Dr. Stevenson after decades of community interventions within Philadelphia, the developers and program coordinator forged a relationship with a local public middle school in West Philadelphia. To establish partnerships, the developers met with school leadership at various points to explain the intervention and understand the needs of the students. When school leadership and the principal investigators mutually agreed, a memorandum of agreement (MOA) was drafted and signed by each party. In one iteration, when school partnerships were not solidified in time for implementation at the start of the school year, we utilized university space within our research lab. In this case, we used this opportunity to recruit families throughout the city, not just within the school with whom we partnered. In expanding our recruitment beyond the families served by our school partner, we were able to diversify our sample with regard to neighborhood composition, socioeconomic status, and educational attainment. With this diversity, we were able to better assess how racial socialization practices vary within different communities.

Partnerships were integral to our recruitment efforts in both iterations. In addition to schools, we sought to partner with and learn from community organizations who were already serving black youth and families in Philadelphia. Our first step was to identify relevant organizations that may be interested in partnering with us. Among these were college readiness programs, churches, youth empowerment groups, and mental health providers. After identifying organizations with whom we were aligned in serving black youth and their families, we developed a succinct document outlining the principles of the intervention, how families benefit (e.g., gift cards, food, and EMBRace "swag"), and how their community organization would benefit (e.g., free clinical services for families within their organization). By providing community partners with a clear, brief overview of how all parties benefitted, we were able to avoid a great deal of confusion. We found that this two-page document integrates well with an MOA if the targeted community organization decides to partner.

In establishing partnerships, we sought out nonprofit organizations and strongholds in our community that are less often involved in research interventions. We believe that as much of the intervention as possible should be community based, even down to the details. For example, in addition to partnering with our local branch of a national college readiness program, the Counseling Department at our university, and local nonprofit organizations, we also partnered with black-owned restaurants to provide the meals we served within our sessions. Our partner was able to give us insight into what meals would be most satisfying for families and the quantities needed for the number of participants we served. Similarly, we were supported by the community in incentivizing the program. A local arcade, based in the community for over forty years, supported our aims and consistently donated arcade vouchers to promote bonding between our EMBRace families outside of sessions. Community-based interventions have the unique opportunity to draw on the strengths of people and organizations who are often excluded from traditional research agendas.

Lessons Learned

(1) Develop an MOA between any community partner and your intervention leadership. (2) Reframe often. What may be considered a setback could be an opportunity to enhance your intervention (or "when life hands you lemons ... "). (3) Expand the idea of partnership to encompass often overlooked members of the community.

Communicating with Scholars, Communities, and Families

Community-based interventions that seek to address health disparities require the passion and effort of various parties toward a common goal. Communicating this shared goal to various stakeholders at universities, within the community, and among the population you hope to serve is a central component to the success of an intervention. Furthermore, interventions have to maintain various forms of communication appropriate for families, researchers, and community partners to garner different types of buy-in (e.g., grant funding, participation, acceptance within organizations, etc.). In the development and implementation of EMBRace, we set systems in place to effectively communicate with researchers, practitioners, community members, and families throughout both iterations of the EMBRace intervention. The EMBRace team has a motto that each product must touch three hands—for example, we must be able to say what we are doing and finding to three different audiences.

EMBRace team members have successfully published three articles: two describing the development and feasibility of the pilot (Anderson et al. 2018a, 2018b), and the other providing a case study (Anderson et al. 2018d) of the initial pilot. We were conscious of the decision to use narrative voice in our publications—thus each manuscript includes language directly from participants to illustrate their experience of discrimination, socialization, and the impact of the program. Team members have attended a variety of conferences and presented findings, workshops, and trainings to demonstrate our procedures. Additionally, we engaged with the community in a variety of ways. We often sought opportunities to interact with organizations at neighborhood or community meetings, and again, prioritized the use of consented visual and auditory aids from our participants when possible. These opportunities in local community organizations within Philadelphia paid respect to the work already being done by families and neighborhoods to fight against racial injustice.

Describing our work to families was likely the most important task for the team. Our goal was to provide an open source of communication to families about the process, progress, and future steps of EMBRace, and we attempted to do this in several ways. First, all contacted families— whether enrolled, interested, or no longer participating—opted into a listserv in which we highlighted local events, family milestones, and opportunities to meet with program staff at community happenings in a monthly newsletter. Second, we utilized social media to highlight relevant articles, media, and spotlights of family participation. Our website also maintains links, pictures, and information pertinent to the intervention. Additionally, we distilled the feasibility findings to a "one-pager," which seeks to clearly and concisely express the findings of the EMBRace pilot study which we provide to families and have linked on our media and web page. Our pamphlets also contain research findings illustrated in relevant examples and culturally grounded depictions of participants.

Two of the most rewarding experiences of the intervention came as a function of meeting with families outside of the seven weeks of the program. A focus group conducted between iterations provided wonderful feedback on client-clinician satisfaction, food choice, and naming conventions (e.g., shifting *homework* to *funwork*). Additionally, a community gathering at the conclusion of the second iteration brought together families to celebrate in their continued success of addressing the challenging task of managing racial stress. The team communicated our findings to the families at the event through a brief report and through individual conversations. These informal experiences were truly helpful in outlining future steps for the program as well as demonstrating the great need of communicating effectively with various stakeholders.

Lessons Learned

(1) Consider which audiences are among the stakeholders for your intervention. What are the ideal methods with which to communicate to these groups? (2) How can you use this opportunity to communicate with different groups to bridge a gap? In communicating with our families, we were able to bring psychoeducation and research findings that are often inaccessible to many EMBRace families. Similarly, the narrative voice used in publications and presentations amplified the needs of our target population. What gaps need to be bridged in your area? (3) Encourage feedback. Each method of communication—whether social media, academic presentation, or community event—allowed for stakeholders to communicate feedback on how to enhance the intervention moving forward.

Reflections from the EMBRace Staff: Why Engage in Community Research?

Within research, reflective practices—in which the researcher should identify the position that they are in with respect to characteristics, desires,

and goals—are critical to the development of community-engaged practices. Communities are systems that require care and maintenance, and
affronts to those systems will often be met with disapproval and frustration for both parties. As such, we wanted to comment on our positionality
as EMBRace team members to discuss in what context our lessons learned
and program development can be understood.

Riana Elyse Anderson, PhD, Principal Investigator/Program Developer

When I was a graduate student in clinical psychology, I grew tired of
reading about the challenges of raising black children. I knew that I was
raised in a loving, supportive, and culturally affirming home in Detroit,
Michigan, and was searching for a representative example of my family
in the literature. Although I eventually found some—most beautifully
illustrated by Dr. Stevenson—I was saddened to see the preponderance
of deficit-based articles on black family life and interventions "fixing"
black people. I was determined at that moment to increase accessibility
and representation within the field of intervention research.

For the advancement of my goals, I had one laser-focused vision:
to join the Racial Empowerment Collaborative at the University of
Pennsylvania to develop a culturally empowered and relevant intervention under the advisement of Dr. Stevenson. After securing a position,
I set out to craft this vision. Two things stand out as most critical to this
story: (1) the buy-in from the community, and (2) the uptake of the intervention by the team.

Upon engaging in my two-year fellowship, my goal was solely to
develop the yet-to-be-named intervention focusing on racial socialization, parenting, and discrimination. After meeting with team members
and getting an outline of the intervention, Dr. Stevenson introduced me

to school leaders, and we discussed the concept of the intervention. They wanted it. I was clear: it was just a concept at this point. They wanted it. I explained that I did not think it would be ready in time. They wanted it. So our team pushed hard to finish the intervention to provide it to the people who we were seeking to serve. It was a labor of love, but ultimately so worth the effort to complete the intervention in time for community implementation.

Second, I never thought in a million years that I would have a team of people who also cared about the vision that I laid out. I was incredibly grateful to be joined by team members after hours, on weekends, or during the summer just to flesh out, implement, and debrief the components of EMBRace. It truly brightens my spirit to know that the next generation of clinicians and researchers may not look in the literature and be displeased—rather, find solutions and data supporting the empowerment and uplifting of black Americans through a clinical intervention started with hope and purpose.

Monique McKenny, MSEd, EMBRace Program Coordinator

Growing up in West Philadelphia, my sister and I received a lot of verbal and nonverbal messages about race. At family dinners on my mother's side, I could identify each and every aforementioned racial socialization tenet within the first thirty minutes of any conversation. Meanwhile, my father's side often communicated through nonverbal messaging. For example, my grandmother would only have black Santa figurines at Christmastime, and when we opened presents, we knew that we would be gifted black Barbie dolls. One Christmas when I was older, she even gifted me a membership to the National Association for the Advancement of Colored People (NAACP).

These racial socialization messages followed me to college and led me to seek out every academic opportunity to better understand the implication of race in the lives of youth. I began pursuing this line of research as an undergraduate and continued post-graduation as I sought further training as a researcher. While in graduate school, I began working with the two principal investigators of EMBRace, Drs. Anderson and Stevenson, at the Racial Empowerment Collaborative. Upon joining the lab, I volunteered for a project that was only described then as a "racial socialization intervention with parents." I was interested in better understanding the factors that influenced how parents socialize their children to race: What experiences had my grandmother had that led her to be so intentional about instilling racial pride, even down to the Christmas decor? How had my sister and I been impacted by the racial socialization messaging we heard in conversations at the dinner table?

While delving into the literature review for EMBRace as a graduate student, I valued the study of racial socialization as a cultural strength. I began to read more literature from scholars who posited racial socialization as a powerful tool that youth and families of color used to protect, empower, and prepare youth in the face of generations of negative racial experiences. Through what I would consider divine orchestration, Drs. Anderson and Stevenson secured a grant that would fund hiring a full-time program coordinator. I was hired, enabling me to continue my work on the intervention. My role as program coordinator allowed me the unique opportunity to work directly with researchers and community leaders, to learn more about clinical training around racial stress, and to witness bonds being strengthened among families from week to week.

At the close of my tenure as program coordinator, I had gained invaluable experience in research and community involvement that has supported me in my continued study of race in the lives of black youth and families. EMBRace gave me insight into how black families are working to prepare their children for the racialized world. Every day, I was able to see how loving caregivers from various backgrounds assembled the tools their children would need to be successful in a society where they would likely experience direct or vicarious encounters with discrimination based on the color of their skin. Within my two years at EMBRace, we worked with families from various socioeconomic backgrounds, religious backgrounds, and family configurations (e.g., adoptive parents, co-parents). The common theme among all of these familial units was the intense love that motivated families to build up their child—to equip, strengthen, and bolster them—toward living happy and healthy lives, much like what was evident in my house growing up.

Conclusion

EMBRace is a novel and needed strategy for reducing racial stress and trauma for both youth and caregivers while increasing family functioning through psychoeducation and the modeling of therapeutic strategies. It is our aim that EMBRace will contribute to social justice on the individual, family, and community levels by alleviating the psychological impact of racialized stress that many black American families and communities carry. It is also our hope that communities can galvanize their resources to support our youth and families for the happy, healthy, and whole units we so desperately desire. Finally, we hope that clinicians, research assistants, and practitioners can develop the skills to best serve our families to restore issues from the past, protect them from racial challenges of today, and build toward a brighter future where racial socialization serves as a strong armor protecting health and well-being.

References

Anderson, R. E., S. B. Hussain, M. N. Wilson, D. S. Shaw, T. J. Dishion, and J. L. Williams. 2015. "Pathways to Pain: Racial Discrimination and Relations between Parental Functioning and Child Psychosocial Well-Being." *Journal of Black Psychology* 41:491–512.

Anderson, R. E., M. McKenny, A. Mitchell, L. Koku, and H. C. Stevenson. 2018a. "EMBRacing Racial Stress and Trauma: Preliminary Feasibility and Coping Responses of a Racial Socialization Intervention." *Journal of Black Psychology* 44:25–46.

Anderson, R. E., M. McKenny, and H. Stevenson. 2018b. "EMBRace: Developing a Racial Socialization Intervention to Reduce Racial Stress and Enhance Racial Coping with Black Parents and Adolescents." *Family Process* 58:53–67.

Anderson, R. E., S. Jones, N. Anwiyo, M. McKenny, and N. Gaylord-Harden. 2018c. "What's Race Got to Do with It? Racial Socialization's Contribution to Black Adolescent Coping." *Journal of Research on Adolescence* 29:822–31.

Anderson, R. E., S. C. Jones, C. C. Navarro, M. C. McKenny, T. J. Mehta, and H. Stevenson. 2018d. "Addressing the Mental Health Needs of Black American Youth and Families: A Case Study from the EMBRace Intervention." *International Journal of Environmental Research and Public Health* 15.

Anderson, R. E., and H. Stevenson. 2016. "EMBRace Training Manual." Unpublished manuscript prepared for the University of Pennsylvania Graduate School of Education's Racial Empowerment Collaborative, Philadelphia.

Anderson, R. E., and H. C. Stevenson. 2019. "RECASTing Racial Stress and Trauma: Theorizing the Healing Potential of Racial Socialization in Families." *American Psychologist* 74, 63.

Belgrave, F. Z., M. C. Reed, L. E. Plybon, and M. Corneille. 2004. "The Impact of a Culturally Enhanced Drug Prevention Program on Drug and Alcohol Refusal Efficacy among Urban African American Girls." *Journal of Drug Education* 34:267–79.

Bowman, P. J., and C. Howard. 1985. "Race-Related Socialization, Motivation, and Academic Achievement: A Study of Black Youths in Three-Generation Families." *Journal of the American Academy of Child Psychiatry* 24:134–41.

Brody, G. H., M. K. Lei, D. H. Chae, T. Yu, S. M. Kogan, and S. R. Beach. 2014. "Perceived Discrimination among African American Adolescents and Allostatic Load: A Longitudinal Analysis with Buffering Effects." *Child Development* 85:989–1002.

Brody, G. H., Y. F. Chen, S. M. Kogan, V. M. Murry, and A. C. Brown. 2010. "Long-Term Effects of the Strong African American Families Program on Youths' Alcohol Use." *Journal of Consulting and Clinical Psychology* 78:281.

Brown, T. N., D. R. Williams, J. S. Jackson, H. W. Neighbors, M. Torres, S. L. Sellers, and K. T. Brown. 2000. "'Being Black and Feeling Blue': The Mental Health Consequences of Racial Discrimination." *Race and Society* 2:117–31.

Burgess, D. J., Y. Ding, M. Hargreaves, M. Van Ryn, and S. Phelan. 2008. "The Association between Perceived Discrimination and Underutilization of Needed Medical and Mental Health Care in a Multi-Ethnic Community Sample." *Journal of Health Care for the Poor and Underserved* 19:894–911.

Carter, R. T. 2007. "Racism and Psychological and Emotional Injury: Recognizing and Assessing Race-Based Traumatic Stress." *Counseling Psychologist* 35:13–105.

Chae, D. H., S. Clouston, M. L. Hatzenbuehler, M. R. Kramer, H. L. Cooper, S. M. Wilson, and B. G. Link. 2015. "Association between an Internet-Based Measure of Area Racism and Black Mortality." *PloS One* 10:e0122963.

Coard, S. I., S. Foy-Watson, C. Zimmer, and A. Wallace. 2007. "Considering Culturally Relevant Parenting Practices in Intervention Development and Adaptation: A Randomized Controlled Trial of the Black Parenting Strengths and Strategies (BPSS) Program." *Counseling Psychologist* 35:797–820.

Harrell, S. P. 2000. "A Multidimensional Conceptualization of Racism-Related Stress: Implications for the Well-Being of People of Color." *American Journal of Orthopsychiatry* 70:42–57.

Harris-Britt, A., C. R. Valrie, B. Kurtz-Costes, and S. J. Rowley. 2007. "Perceived Racial Discrimination and Self-Esteem in African American Youth: Racial Socialization as a Protective Factor." *Journal of Research on Adolescence* 17:669–82.

Hughes, D., J. Rodriguez, E. P. Smith, D. J. Johnson, H. C. Stevenson, and P. Spicer. 2006. "Parents' Ethnic-Racial Socialization Practices: A Review of Research and Directions for Future Study." *Developmental Psychology* 42:747.

Hughes, D., D. Witherspoon, D. Rivas-Drake, and N. West-Bey. 2009. "Received Ethnic–Racial Socialization Messages and Youths' Academic and Behavioral Outcomes: Examining the Mediating Role of Ethnic Identity and Self-Esteem." *Cultural Diversity and Ethnic Minority Psychology* 15:112.

Jones, S. C., and E. W. Neblett. 2016. "Racial–Ethnic Protective Factors and Mechanisms in Psychosocial Prevention and Intervention Programs for Black Youth." *Clinical Child and Family Psychology Review* 19:134–61.

Lesane-Brown, C. L. 2006. "A Review of Race Socialization within Black Families." *Developmental Review* 26:400–26.

Metzger, I. W., T. Salami, S. Carter, C. Halliday-Boykins, R. E. Anderson, M. M. Jernigan, and T. Ritchwood. 2018. "African American Emerging Adults' Experiences with Racial Discrimination and Drinking Habits: The Moderating Roles of Perceived Stress." *Cultural Diversity and Ethnic Minority Psychology* 24:489.

National Public Radio (NPR), Robert Wood Johnson Foundation (RWJF), and Harvard University T. H. Chan School of Public Health. 2017. *Discrimination in America: Experiences and Views of African Americans*. Princeton, NJ: Robert Wood Johnson Foundation.

Neblett Jr., E. W., T. M. Chavous, H. X. Nguyên, and R. M. Sellers. 2009. "'Say It Loud—I'm Black and I'm Proud': Parents' Messages about Race, Racial Discrimination, and Academic Achievement in African American Boys." *Journal of Negro Education*, 246–59.

Neblett, E. W., C. L. Philip, C. D. Cogburn, and R. M. Sellers. 2006. "African American Adolescents' Discrimination Experiences and Academic Achievement: Racial Socialization as a Cultural Compensatory and Protective Factor." *Journal of Black Psychology* 32:199–218.

Neblett, E. W., C. P. Smalls, K. R. Ford, H. X. Nguyen, and R. M. Sellers. 2009. "Racial Socialization and Racial Identity: African American Parents' Messages about Race as Precursors to Identity." *Journal of Youth and Adolescence* 38:189–203.

Neff, K. D. 2003. "The Development and Validation of a Scale to Measure Self-Compassion." *Self and Identity* 2:223–50.

Pachter, L., B. Bernstein, L. Szalacha, and C. Coll. 2010. "Perceived Racism and Discrimination in Children and Youths: An Exploratory Study." *Health & Social Work* 35:61–69.

Seaton, E. K., G. H. Caldwell, R. M. Sellers, and J. S. Jackson. 2010. "An Intersectional Approach for Understanding Perceived Discrimination and Psychological Well-Being among African American and Caribbean Black Youth." *Developmental Psychology* 46:1372.

Slopen, N., T. T. Lewis, and D. R. Williams. 2016. "Discrimination and Sleep: a Systematic Review." *Sleep Medicine* 18:88–95.

Stevenson, H. C., ed. 2003. *Playing with Anger: Teaching Coping Skills to African American Boys through Athletics and Culture*. Westport, CT: Greenwood Publishing Group.

Stevenson, H. C. 2014. *Promoting Racial Literacy in Schools: Differences That Make a Difference*. New York: Teachers College Press.

Wang, M., and J. P. Hughley. 2012. "Parental Racial Socialization as a Moderator of the Effects of Racial Discrimination among African American Adolescents." *Child Development* 83:1716–31.

Williams, D. R., and S. A. Mohammed. 2009. "Discrimination and Racial Disparities in Health: Evidence and Needed Research." *Journal of Behavioral Medicine* 32:20–47.

Williams, D. R., H. W. Neighbors, and J. S. Jackson. 2003. "Racial/Ethnic Discrimination and Health: Findings from Community Studies." *American Journal of Public Health* 93:200–08.

Chapter 7

Rebuilding Affrilachia

DeWayne Barton
Hood Huggers International

Chapter Context

I was born into community work. My father was very active in the neighbor-hood and showed me at a young age the importance of doing things within the community, including how to develop relationships between youth and the adults. I definitely hated it, particularly on Saturday mornings when I wanted to be playing with my friends. As an adult, I can look back now and appreciate the gift of being the youngest person sitting in those community meetings and being the "gopher"—go for this, go for that! My father's words and actions, as well as the elders, taught me about collaboration and how working together makes a community thrive.

Hood Huggers International exists to create opportunities within histori-cally marginalized communities for its members to gain knowledge, learn skills and trades, and become entrepreneurs, all of which give back to and sustain the community. Our goal is to restore our neighborhoods and to build them back to the loving environment where we lifted each other up and supported one another—to gain what we lost before the introduction of crack cocaine. Hood

Huggers International realizes that people cannot sustain themselves wading in a pool with only one foot of water when we can design one that is thirteen feet deep; people can safely jump in and go a lot further.

Hood Huggers International's focuses primarily on arts, the environment, and social enterprise. The arts, including visual and performative art, serve as a creative outlet for individual expression and healing. We look to the environment to provide us with a reflective and conscious lens for rebuilding connection. Engaging the community in social enterprise allows us to uplift and celebrate our collaborative work and to grow individually and collectively.

On every tour, patrons engage with the history of Asheville, North Carolina, and are educated about what has been lost over the years. Tour income is not only reinvested in the business—Hood Huggers International maintains and supports additional programming like experiential classes on collaborative networking and team building and the Peace Garden. We have also supplied startup capital for grassroots organizations, MS Lean Landscaping and Green Opportunities. Lastly, we are able to further our research in identifying, protecting, and securing infrastructure within our community.

What we are realizing is that the trauma and pain in our community runs deep, preventing collaborative connections. We now know that we have to go even deeper to get to the root and heal those wounds. It will truly take local grassroots efforts to effect the changes that we'd like to see. While there are many well-intentioned organizations that are doing great work in our communities, the challenges that have been targeted for improvement still exist. We suggest that these external influences are not always community driven, often operate on perceived notions of community needs, or are motivated by funding priorities, all of which ultimately exacerbate the divide.

We intend to create a new pattern in our neighborhoods that operates on what the community identifies as its priorities, and then we will match those needs to already existing and newly developed programs led by community members. We will solicit and obtain external resources to grow and expand strong community initiatives and to support redevelopment. We would act as liaison and encourage partnerships with outside institutions that create systems and have the ability to put mechanisms in place that will support, educate, and train individuals to continue the work on their own.

Introduction

As a young man, the US Navy gave me the opportunity to see many parts of the world. At the age of thirty-three, I determined that I would return to traveling and exploring other cultures, either in the Peace Corps or as a civilian contractor, not in the navy. One day, my mother called and said that she wanted me to leave Norfolk and head back to Asheville. My instant reaction to that request was a resounding no! There was nothing in Asheville for me except my mother and other family members. I tried to understand her perspective though; my father and aunt had recently died and my mother needed me. There really was no option. I resolved to return home for maybe six months, maybe a year, to see if I could help my mother settle in again after the loss of our loved ones. I headed back to Burton Street.

My family had moved from Asheville to Washington, DC, when I was a young man, so I was raised in the city. I always loved our frequent trips to Asheville to be with family. In Asheville I experienced country life with woods and neighborhoods that felt safe and warm to me after the fast-paced life of DC. Things were changing in DC with the advent of drugs and violence. On returning to Asheville after a number of years, I was shocked to find that the same self-destructive forces that had torn areas around DC apart were at work here on Burton Street. The health of the community was being destroyed.

I looked around at mountains of discarded needles, homemade crack pipes, forty-ounce liquor bottles, cans, lighters, and piles of garbage. There was an open-air drug market in place that literally regulated the flow of traffic in the neighborhood. I couldn't help but think about the destruction drugs brought to my DC community, and was afraid the same thing was happening to my Burton Street neighborhood. Families were destroyed, the land value dropped, and prisons were full. This was a reality for so many young and impressionable people with limited opportunities.

How I Got Started

One morning, a short time after my return home, I stepped outside my house and ended up between two guys shooting at each other. It was a profoundly sobering moment. I decided then that I was going to try something to help restore the health of my community. When I was a child and, later, during my teen years in DC, my stepfather had worked extensively in our community; as a result, I spent a great deal of time working with him, and I hated it. I didn't think working with my step-father was cool. Determined to avoid facing armed drug dealers, I began to wonder what I could do that would be a relatively safe enterprise. I looked around the neighborhood and again saw the immense piles of garbage and decided to start by simply picking up trash. When I was twelve years old, I started my own small business collecting cans, so this was not new to me. Additionally, this was something that would not be perceived as threatening to anyone in the neighborhood. This may sound like a small and insignificant task, but it was a safe place to start.

For a very long time, I was alone in my endeavors. Neighbors would peer at me through closed windows. They began looking for me, wanting to see if I would continue what seemed like an overwhelming and point-less task considering the other more pressing problems the neighborhood had, so I continued my work. It took several years of picking up trash, day after day, before the neighbors began to realize the depth of my com-mitment and started connecting with others who wanted to help. Folks began to open up to me then. At that point, we began to pay young people to join our efforts and help.

I had been totally unaware that mothers in the neighborhood started the Burton Street Advisory Committee in 1967, the year I was born, and had been meeting regularly since then. My mother showed me a news-paper article that had a photograph of more than two hundred women marching on Haywood Road, the main road that runs through West Asheville. The neighborhood mothers were marching, trying to bring attention to the issues of the Burton Street neighborhood in 1992. I was humbled. The mothers had a long history of hard work in trying to save the neighborhood from the war on drugs.

Burton Street was founded in 1912 by E. W. Pearson, a veteran of the Spanish-American War, and founder of the first North Carolina chapter of the National Association for the Advancement of Colored People (NAACP). It was a self-sustaining, culturally enforced, segregated, African American community. There was a nursing school, several busi-nesses, and a Negro League baseball team. There was an annual agricul-tural fair that drew more than fifteen thousand people, both black and white, to the neighborhood. There was a strong emphasis on education and universal support for the elementary school. It was a strong, healthy, thriving community.

Urban Renewal began in Asheville in the 1950s and continued into the 1970s. It was the largest urban renewal project in the Southeast. Over four hundred acres of black homes and businesses were lost throughout the city. The Burton Street neighborhood was decimated by the widen-ing of Patton Avenue in the 1950s and, later in the 1960s, I-240 further fragmented the community. Roots were being ripped out and many prominent families moved away, leaving a vacuum.

This urban renewal led to the thirty-year war on drugs. The overall health of the community was interrupted. The great reputation and connection of the community were lost. How does a community rebuild itself from the inside out? We continued our revitalization efforts in the neighborhood. One day the City of Asheville sent a representative to one of our community meetings and informed us that they had plans to close the community center under the pretext of budgetary considerations and the drug problem. This helped galvanize the community. We convinced the youth to get involved working to help save the center to start writing letters, and even a song, to the city, state, and federal officials. The youth sang, "We going down if Burton Street is not around. Our whole life will be turned upside down" at neighborhood meetings and during a city council meeting in order to get people to support the effort. Elders and young people went to the city council, and our combined efforts paid off. The city decided to keep the center open.

Capitalizing on our momentum, we took our actions further and asked for help renovating the center and other neighborhood improvements. Officials came out to the neighborhood and walked around, looking at things like the antiquated heating system and kitchen. We continued with our clean up and the renovations to the community center. During this time, I was working at the Youth Development Center (YDC), essen-tially a youth prison. Looking back, this was a crossroad in my life. I spent my days at the YDC teaching these young men. In the evening, I returned home to witness the environmental conditions that helped send them there. They weren't being taught; they were just being held there.

I began to get creative with the youth. In the lobby of the building was a snack machine. Getting something from this snack machine was a very big deal for the youth, so I bargained with them. I went to Prison Books in Asheville and picked up a wide assortment of books. They were free, and I would take them to the YDC with me. When one of the kids would ask me if I would get him something from the snack machine, I would say, "Sure if you'll read one of these books and write about it—no less than two pages and no more than five pages—I will certainly get you a snack." The youth didn't spend a lot of time reading so I was trying to get them engaged. It was a wild success. I still have hundreds of these book reports from the young people. Later, I began paying them for the artwork they produced in their art classes to encourage them to practice creative expression through the arts. It became very apparent to me that the community is the headwater in society. They go to school to practice what they're taught at home and in the neighborhood. I was in a position between my work in the Burton Street community and my work at the YDC to clearly see the connection between lack of support and poor infrastructure and how that led to an increased number of young people going to prison. Once I realized this, I left the YDC and began to focus on the neighborhood with renewed efforts.

The Peace Garden

I met my wife, Safi, when she came around to help clean up the neighborhood. She was an activist in her own right, trying to prevent a Walmart from being built in a historical area of Asheville. She was also environmentally aware, and we had much in common. We moved into our home on Burton Street. One day Safi walked around the neighborhood, came back to the house, and said, "Let's make a garden." We named it the

Peace Garden because of the war in Iraq and the war on drugs in our neighborhood; we did it in order to draw people out of their homes to interact with each other and build relationships. We would make art out of trash we collected and would also grow food. We focused on our neighborhood. We developed relationships with schools and communities to help maintain it. The garden, a labor of love, lies in the heart of the Burton Street community. From its humble beginnings as an overgrown lot filled with trash, the gardens have grown to include two vegetable/flower gardening sites, a staging area, a fire pit, a cob pizza oven, a greenhouse, a pavilion, a store, paintings, sculptures, and a composting toilet.

With a focus on environmental and community responsibility, the garden design and sculpture park have been created using found/reused items mostly from the immediate neighborhood. The gardens are hydrated using direct rain, in addition to rainwater collected in the 550-gallon tank of a neighboring residence. The greenhouse frame was constructed using steel poles from a discarded McDonald's playground. Brick, block, and concrete used to build the fire pit, garden beds, and cob oven are all sourced from residences or sidewalks that were demolished and headed for the landfill. The 300-square-foot pavilion, which serves as a gathering space and teaching tool for the neighborhood and beyond, is also made of many salvaged and repurposed materials. Of special note is the sculpture park, which is the creative endeavor of a lot of local artists, myself included. The installations are created with found/reused items, and each tells a separate and compelling story of social and environmental justice and black history.

The goal of the Peace Garden was to establish infrastructure and relationships that would allow health-related programs to occur. We distribute organic vegetables to elders and help others grow and maintain their own gardens. We have a pizza oven that is used for special events. In the community, we provide a free space for people to visit—school groups, tourists—and we hold special events to bring diverse people together. It is used for community service projects. We allow environmental and social justice groups to meet in the garden. We use it for training space for young and adult people who need to learn more about business and gardening.

The Burton Street Peace Gardens have, over the years, become a sanctuary for positive action, designed to create neighborhood food security, community cohesion, and a vibrant, sustainable local economy. Every spring and fall we hold plant and flower sales, so neighbors can have plants to start their own gardens. There is a donation bin near the garden gate with a sign that reads: "Take what you need, leave what you can." This way people without gardens have access to homegrown vegetables, and they often leave money to contribute to the refurbishment of our garden. Several times a year we have neighborhood parties where we cook vegetables or pizzas and have live music from the neighborhood to continue to engage with the people around the city. The pavilion is used as a classroom. It is also available for meeting space. There is a library so that people in the neighborhood have access to reading material.

After our initial success, the city applied for, and received, the federal Weed and Seed grant. The point was to "weed" out the drugs and "seed" the neighborhood. We had been working to find more sustainable ways to pay the kids and adults for their work in the community. They were able to obtain this grant because of the work that we had already been doing in the neighborhood. Unfortunately 70 percent of the funding went to policing the neighborhood and only 30 percent came to the neighborhood itself. Safi and I had been paying the kids to help with the work in the neighborhood, but when so little of the funding from the Weed and Seed grant came through, we began to look for more sustainable ways to pay

the kids. The money received from the grant was used to build the neighborhood entrance sign. The young people in the neighborhood built the
sign and were trained in skills of painting, woodworking, and design.
The men in the neighborhood helped with the training and the sign was
built. I realized then that we needed to start a program around training
young men with skills. This project provided the impetus for a landscaping business and Green Opportunities, a green jobs training program.

Asheville Green Opportunities

Later, I was very excited to attend a conference on the state of black
Asheville—held at University of North Carolina, Asheville. This UNC
project does research about differences along racial lines in terms of
healthcare, business, criminal justice, and education in Asheville. I
wanted to be able to share and learn about other neighborhood efforts
and how we might connect. But at the conference, I learned the issues
were greater than I imagined. The historical background and current
conditions as presented made me realize just how widespread and monumental the issues were. I left the conference angry and went to a play
at the Edington Center and watched a performance that showed a lot of
young people believing that they had a future in this city. I was still upset
from what I had learned at the conference and realized I had to go harder
and larger.

I focused on a plan to be able to train young people in trade skills that
were environmentally friendly. I spoke to many people about this idea;
those who knew about solar, weatherization, and building in an environmentally conscious way. I found that nothing existed for training young
people in green skills that would be focused in their neighborhoods. The
idea for Green Opportunities (GO) was born. In my youth, I had gone

through a similar training program to learn trade skills like masonry, carpentry, plumbing, and electricity, but the program was poorly run, which is how I ended up in the navy. With Green Opportunities, I knew that we could make the neighborhood the school itself. We could recruit youth from the neighborhood, help them acquire trade skills with a specific environmental focus (thus *green* opportunities). The goal would be for the kids to advance from obtaining their GED's to establishing trade skills, and then go on to become entrepreneurs, inventors, or to seek advancement in school. There was a lot of creativity in youth that had yet to be tapped. Additionally, it was equally critical that we engage with workers and business leaders in the community, so we could build a lasting base for training these young people.

We began training young people to be more environmentally conscious in their own neighborhoods. We weatherized churches, homes, and all public housing units in Asheville, using people who lived there to do it. We were recruiting young men and women who had been convicted of felonies, training them, and giving them skill sets to do the work. Engagement was the most important part of GO. We had to involve these young people because they were only going to be in the program for a period of six months to a year.

With help from co-founder Dan Leroy, we began canvassing and recruiting businesses in the Asheville area that would commit to supporting our Green Opportunities program. From these beginnings, Green Opportunities built an energy team that performs home energy audits and basic weatherization services for private clients. It has grown into a healthy fee-for-service program and is now an apprentice host for others in the program. Other apprentice hosts include FLS Energy, Sundance Power Systems, Winter Green, and the Asheville Housing Authority. The Asheville City Council approved the housing and community development plan, which included approximately $162,000 in funding for Asheville GO across two categories: construction and nonconstruction. Along with the green energy program, Green Opportunities also renovated the Arthur R. Edington Education and Career Center, a multimillion-dollar project. The center was located in a low-income neighborhood and would be used to house Green Opportunities training, academic enrichment, after-school programs, and other community events. Partners in this project included the City of Asheville, the Western North Carolina Green Building Council, AB Technical College, the Empowerment Resource Center of Asheville, the Asheville Housing Authority, the YWCA, Mountain Bizworks, area churches, neighborhood associations, and community groups. The Peace Garden green space is a place for healing. It is an incubator—it cultivates other things like the GO job training program and protecting the neighborhood community center, et cetera. A community accountability plan (CAP) is the formula to start and maintain these community programs. GO is currently set to start renovation on the theatre in the Edington Building. The Edington Center holds offices for GO, the housing authority, and academic enrichment activities, including an after-school program. GO Kitchen already serves lunch, and people come together for a meal. People in the training program are paid with donations from members of the community. Once a year there is a fundraising dinner, and everyone is invited.

Green Opportunities celebrated its tenth year in 2018. Now I'm the president of the Burton Street Community Association. We were told that the highway project that was proposed several years earlier was back on the table and the neighborhood was going to take a significant blow like others from the past. We were shocked after all the work, relationship building, and sacrifice. One night at a Department of Transportation (DOT) meeting in the neighborhood, I asked the local executive director from the Asheville Design Center for help. Can you help create our own neighborhood plan, a plan we could give to the DOT to honor? If you're going take over 160 homes and businesses, we want you to honor our plan by lessening your impact and investing back into our community. We attended thousands of meetings, marches, and interviews. The process of creating a neighborhood plan was intense, but everyone was talking about "Save Burton Street." We later found out our community was designated as an environmental justice community. They will have to invest back into our neighborhood. We began in 2009 with help from students from Appalachian State University. Despite door-to-door survey and group meetings that led to a finished plan in 2010, it collected dust. In 2018 it was finally adopted by the city but with no timeline or budget. Our goal now is to make the plan come alive by expanding on existing infrastructure.

The Community Accountability Plan

These experiences led to the creation of Hood Huggers International, a social enterprise designed to heal, rebuild, and sustain historically marginalized communities. We would use the profits from Hood Tours to help restore the neighborhoods we visit. All our lives we've heard about tree huggers and how they chain themselves to trees to prevent their destruction, and I knew I felt that way about my neighborhood, thus Hood Huggers International was born.

I designed the community accountability plan (CAP). It's a framework designed to assist others in similar activities. I wanted to put together a plan that would hold people, both in the neighborhood and in the surrounding communities, accountable for the commitments they make to sustain community health and growth. I wanted to highlight the importance of building a pipeline of support and creating a platform via practice.

We live in an atmosphere of historical trauma, which makes it hard to build on united strengths. It is important to create an atmosphere where gaps in service can be filled and existing services can be made stronger. We struggle to connect and build while maintaining trusting regenerative relationships. CAP is based on trial, error, and success—a ground-up learning experience. It is challenging to get support, but this is crucial. CAP can provide a framework to connect the dots and build capacity. It helps with filtering out people or businesses that say they want to commit, but never follow up. CAP has an internal and external framework design and flowcharts that help identify and weed out the unnecessary complications. This is a way to implement and celebrate grassroots revitalization and accountability. It is a system designed to build, maintain, and protect pillars of resiliency in historically African American neighborhoods. The CAP supports a culture of sustainability that is inclusive and economically just. The plan also includes creating, maintaining, and connecting green spaces that help absorb trauma.

The state of black Asheville conference was part of the fuel that led to the creation of CAP. In a public policy course at the University of North Carolina, Asheville, which Dr. Dwight Mullen has been teaching since 2006, students pick a topic of interest and study the influence race has on local public policy. Afterward, they share their findings with the public. With CAP, businesses, nonprofits, community volunteers, and government agencies operate in response to the plans of neighborhood leaders, working to implement their vision for their communities rather than prescribing solutions or programs. The three key components of CAP are the arts, the environment, and social enterprise. With community capacity building, we utilize some community engagement tools such as interactive storytelling, community coaches, neighborhood beautification projects, inclusive community events, resources, and education. One example of this is our development of a neighborhood-based Youth Credit Union where young people can practice financial literacy. The kids are paid for their work and then offered an opportunity to have their money matched should they choose to set up a savings account. We have a current working relationship with Self Help Credit Union, a local-based credit union in Asheville.

A large issue has been connecting city policy with action on the ground. Working with Green Opportunities, the Peace Garden, and other projects gives one the ability to see how all the working parts could come together, but it's difficult to get groups to work together. Commitment and connection are vital. The City of Asheville has developed a comprehensive plan, the Disparity Study, which aims to assess whether minority and women-owned businesses face any barriers in the city's contracting processes. The city also has a Human Relations Council and a gentrification study in place. Another one is the I-26 Connector Project, which will seriously affect the Burton Street community. My vision, as far as the community accountability plan goes, is to ensure that the city is working with individuals and businesses from the neighborhood. This will facilitate a healthy working relationship with many different perspectives taken into consideration to achieve the various goals set in each of these initiatives. The goal of the CAP is to connect the neighborhood with the city's various plans and programs to build a culture of community accountability and relationship building to ensure that the community works together to maintain health and growth.

Hood Huggers and the Hood Tours

I thought about the importance of our history in Asheville. I wanted to find a way to share that past and help inspire the future. Black history was obscure in this city. So much so, in fact, that areas of important black historical significance were being erased. The black hospital, located in what is now part of the South Slope Brewery area, is now a parking lot for tourists. The E. W. Pearson Building, once located on Burton Street, is now gone. Seeing tour buses flying through the black neighborhoods, I wondered to myself, *How are they talking about the black neighborhoods?* I went to visit the chamber of commerce. There, I was told by a local tour company there was no real interest in the black history. They told me that if I wrote up a synopsis, they would give them to their drivers. I tried writing the script, but thought, *No. I'm going to do this myself.* I wanted this to not only be about informing people about the history but also the current health of these places. They needed to understand what it means to tear down neighborhood landmarks. The cultural history is rich here. I wanted to highlight the history and protect what was left of our landmarks. Entire neighborhoods were obliterated, and Allen High School, the only school for African American women, saw E. W. Pearson's two daughters through their curriculum as well as Nina Simone. We still have Triangle Park and the Stephens-Lee Community Center. We still have the YMI Cultural Center, one of the oldest in the country. If we don't talk about our spaces and people, they will be lost in memories. These communities make an art out of making a way forward. The Stephens-Lee Alumni Association is trying to turn what is left of the school into a museum. The Hood Tours works to support organizations that are already doing the work to save these places. The county has now allocated funds for historical markers to be displayed, and tourism and development have allocated over $100,000 to assist with the creation of a museum in the Stephens-Lee Auditorium.

Conclusion

These days I spend my time giving tours to both locals who want to learn about the black history this city holds, and to tourists coming in from all over the world. The tours support nonprofit groups and businesses who are trying to rebuild the community, I give guest copies of the *Hood Huggers Green Book*, highlighting current black-owned businesses and nonprofits that are helping rebuild the community in Asheville. The *Hood Huggers Green Book* is loosely modeled after the *Negro Motorist Green Book* that was published for many years by Victor Green, directing traveling African Americans to friendly businesses, restaurants, and hotels in the Jim Crow era. We want to show people where and how to connect today, right now, with black-owned businesses. We talk about the resilient economic history of the past, current conditions, and how we can rebuild a stronger future together.

I then take my visitors to the Peace Garden to wander through the vegetables, flowers, and sculptures to soak in the serenity and creativity that emanates from that wonderful space. When I am not touring, I divide my time between the neighborhood, city hall, and the surrounding community, looking to fill gaps and holes where I find them; shoring up the foundation of what we continue to build in Asheville, a healthy environment for growth and creativity.

If you really want to build a healthy and flourishing environment for your community, start with picking up trash and building a garden.

Chapter 8

The Evolution of Health and Housing for One Community-Based Organization

Robert Torres
The Urban Edge

Chapter Context

Before working in affordable housing and community development I focused on policy issues as they related to mental health and substance abuse. What became extremely evident during this time was that housing is a major barrier to people achieving positive health outcomes. As my career transitioned into housing and community development I began to better understand health issues in Boston and how closely tied they are to historic government actions, such as redlining and housing discrimination. At Urban Edge we have been quite proud of the work we have done, but we realized that we need to be intentional about driving positive health outcomes. We know that health inequities exist, the racial wealth gap is real, and the life expectancy gap is something we need to address—but are we really having a positive impact with the work that we are doing, and can we have greater impact?

At Urban Edge, we provide affordable housing and supportive services to residents. Traditionally we have created programs in response to needs in the community. For years we have been proud of the programs and housing we have created, but, historically, we have not approached this work with a health lens. We recognize that some people may just need a home, then they can afford to live a healthy life. Others require a host of services that run along a continuum—from very basic needs, such as connection or information about resources, to more holistic support services. Urban Edge's services have typically fallen in the front half of the continuum and have not been at the back end, which would include assisted living. Still, we know now that our housing and services have been impacting health, but have we established a culture of health?

What we learned throughout this project is that affordable housing and intentionally designed programs make people healthier. In many ways, however, we already knew this, and we have known this for a long time. Over the years we have become increasingly data informed, data driven, and evidence based in an effort to prove our impact. For smaller organizations these data-driven practices are very costly and take up a significant portion of staff time. So after we have proven what we already knew—that affordable housing and services positively impact health—we have to ask ourselves: Have we increased our impact? For me, the data piece is very important, but we should use data systems to help increase our impact in the community, not take focus away from the mission of our organization.

Introduction

New York, San Francisco, Silicon Valley, and Boston are the four most expensive housing markets in the United States (Walsh, Doyle, and Valdes Lupi 2018). The pressures that high rents and overall housing costs put on Boston's residents became increasingly clear to me while working for a member of the Massachusetts state legislature. From 2009

to 2014 I worked for an elected official whose top priority was addressing issues that pertain to mental health and substance abuse. During this
time, it became troubling to see how difficult life can be when trying to
address a serious health issue while struggling to pay for housing.

During my five years working for the Massachusetts House of
Representatives, I was connected to hundreds of people who sincerely
wanted to improve their health but struggled to afford housing. It became
clear that housing was an essential part of living a healthy life, and I
wanted to be part of the solution. In 2014 I made the decision to transition to a community-based organization that focuses on building quality
affordable housing, Urban Edge Community Development Corporation.
Moving to an affordable housing organization after working for a state
legislator seemed like a natural progression. After seeing how the cost of
housing causes people to forego important health needs, such as seeking
treatment for substance abuse, I wanted to work for an organization that
would be intentional in building a culture of health. An organization that
thinks about health throughout all their practices, not just traditional
health services, but a general understanding that all our interactions with
clients can potentially impact their health. An organization that understands that not all people have equal opportunities to lead healthier lives.

Urban Edge was founded in 1974 as a response to the effects of redlining, displacement, and real estate speculation on low-income residents.
Members of the community organized in response to the state's plan to
extend I-95 through the neighborhood and began bringing the community back from "the urban edge." In the mid-1970s Urban Edge began
acquiring vacant and foreclosed properties and put them back into use,
shaping the path toward a robust affordable housing stock with a focus
on community development. Forty years later, when I joined the organization, they had a portfolio of over 1,300 units of affordable housing

and 100,000 square feet of retail and community space. It has been widely written about how these phenomena that drove the creation of Urban Edge also had lasting effects on segregation in schools as well as in neighborhoods.

At Urban Edge, I oversee a group of professionals who provide a host of services to residents. Our support services focus on the areas of housing stability, financial capabilities, and leadership development. The average wait time to move into an Urban Edge property is six years. It is our philosophy that if a family endured the waitlist process, we as an organization need to ensure that a family has the opportunity to live in stable housing and prosper. Residents are "housing stable" when they can afford their rent and live without feeling at risk of being evicted. Using the culture of health framework that the Robert Wood Johnson Foundation has developed, we are now on a mission to improve our services and programs in ways that will drive improved health, well-being, and equity.

Making Health a Shared Value

In 2014 Urban Edge put together a strategic plan that is designed to guide the organization from 2015 through 2020. The strategic planning process involved Urban Edge's staff, board members, residents, and other community stakeholders. One of the outcomes of the strategic planning process was that health and wellness were identified as core values for the organization. Health was a key driver of what will strengthen residents, families, and, ultimately, our community.

Through this strategic planning process, health was officially declared a shared value, authorizing our organization to begin an evolution that would set our mindset and expectations about how we, as a community-based organization, can better impact the health of our residents through our housing and services. In addition to health, education was identified as an opportunity area for our residents. The idea that emerged during the strategic planning process was that if low-income people had homes they could afford, there would be more time and resources available to address health and educational needs.

Health and Housing 1.0: Cross-Sector Collaboration

In 2015 we decided to expand a budding pre-K readiness program created a year earlier using a resident-driven process. Through a series of focus groups, interviews, and surveys, residents identified several educational programs they wanted to participate in but were unable to attend due to the program location or conflicting schedules. The feedback led us to design a program that has classes two nights a week with educational opportunities for parents and their children. We were able to successfully expand this program by forming new collaborations with a local health partner and a new technology partner. The partners who worked together to create this program were Families First, JumpStart, Baraka Community Wellness, and Union Capital Boston.

Families First is our program partner who works collaboratively with us to help parents increase their parenting skills, knowledge, and support systems. During the time that parents interact with Families First, a greater Boston-based organization, children ages three to five are able to build academic and social skills necessary for success with JumpStart, an early learning provider who has programming in fourteen states (including Washington, DC).

Residents also called for a health component, citing that eating healthy food was expensive and opportunities to exercise were difficult to work into an already busy schedule. To solve our health programming needs we partnered with a local health organization, Baraka Community Wellness, which offers health coaching, physical fitness, nutrition, and cooking demonstrations. Baraka Community Wellness also offers access to fresh produce.

After identifying partners in different sectors to help us with our programming needs, we took our first step into health and housing by working with a cohort of twenty parents and their children. We measured hours spent exercising, hours in self-care, time spent reading with their children, and pounds of healthy food distributed to families each week. Parents reported that they played with their children more, used better communication skills, felt more connected to their neighbors, and used positive reinforcement more often. We were able to track these outcomes with the help of another collaborator, Union Capital Boston, a smartphone rewards app that allows members to earn points that accumulate to cash rewards by checking in to civic engagement and volunteer opportunities such as pre-K readiness programs, or time spent reading to their children.

This program was our first intervention that included health as a dimension in addition to our educational goals. Exercise and healthy eating are activities we want to encourage in the community, but how should a community-based housing organization create a culture of health? Realizing the success of this program, we decided to explore other paths that might contribute to a culture of health—a culture that allows every Urban Edge resident to access healthy food, feel safe, breathe quality air, and, above all, have more equitable opportunities to live healthier lives.

Health and Housing 2.0: The Nexus of Health and Housing?

At Urban Edge, we often spoke about health and housing as a nexus, some sort of intersection where the two eventually cross. Our thinking was that if we could identify that point of intersection, we might be able to have a meaningful impact on individual and community health. In 2016 we began to form a new program with a well-known mobile health clinic, the Family Van. This partnership was a literal attempt to connect housing with healthcare. We began by collecting data from residents to learn more about their perceptions about health needs in the community. Data we collected also helps us better understand where community residents receive their health services and the health issues residents see in the community. Ultimately we wanted to know if residents would be amenable to participating in health-related programs that take place at Urban Edge; the survey results informed us that they would.

Recently there have been numerous publications that describe housing as a key driver of health outcomes. Still, funders have looked for programs that highlight successful health and housing partnerships that further prove this correlation. Urban Edge and the Family Van designed a program in the hopes of proving that our affordable housing, coupled with our programs and services, has a positive impact on the health of our residents. To do this, we needed the health and research expertise of the Family Van. The Family Van helped craft a new-move-in program that largely relied on a health impact questionnaire (HIQ) that was designed to measure the impact that Urban Edge's housing and services had on residents.

Utilizing Cross-Sector Collaborators: Leveraging Expertise

When we were first working with the Family Van, we were asked to describe which of our services were health related. As we were trying to answer this question it became very clear to our partner that looking at our services and residents with a health lens was new for us. Through a mapping exercise with the entire community engagement team, we were able to map out exactly which services where directly health related, indirectly health related, and which were not health related.

As a housing provider, we at Urban Edge take pride in the quality of our affordable housing and range of services. Some of the services we offer include financial coaching, leadership development, eviction prevention, student loan counseling, benefits enrollment, free tax preparation, summer youth jobs, first-time home buyer classes, and connection to resources. Typically we have measured our impact in terms of degree of financial impact. For example, if we connect someone to $300 worth of Supplemental Nutrition Assistance Program (SNAP) benefits each month, and their monthly income is $1,000, we have determined that their income has increased by 30 percent. Since 2012 Urban Edge has connected residents to $1.2 million in means-tested government benefits, of which nearly $500,000 was in SNAP benefits. Traditionally we would have seen the increase in income strictly as a financial gain; however, we now understand that SNAP is linked to health improvements in current and long-term health (Carlson and Keith-Jennings 2018).

Now that we have a better understanding of how our services address the social determinants of health, we put together a plan that we thought would test our hypothesis.

Hypothesis: *Urban Edge's impact on housing and financial stability; access to quality housing they can afford, coupled with financial stability services and* *better access to healthcare; will have positive impacts on health, both in terms of intermediary health measures and longer-term health outcomes.*

The Plan

- Work with property management to identify new move-ins. Urban Edge owns 1,350 units of affordable housing; however, we outsource all property management functions to a third-party private property management company.

- Have a member of the Urban Edge Community Engagement team meet with new residents within one month of moving into their apartment. Urban Edge outsources property management functions but has kept resident services in-house and rebranded the department as Community Engagement.

- Offer all Urban Edge services to new move-ins, track the services that families are connected to, and, most importantly, build a relationship with the resident/families who move in. The relationship between the Community Engagement team and residents is core to Urban Edge's philosophy that resident services are a means to community building and engagement.

- Begin to build a relationship in the first visit by getting to know the new move-in on a personal level. Conduct a benefit screening for means-tested government benefits, offer financial coaching services, and administer the ten-question health impact questionnaire.

- Incentivize the new residents to visit the Family Van for a health screening. As an incentive to visit the van, residents were provided with two movie passes after completing their initial health screening. The purpose of the health screening was to gather a baseline of biometric health data, including BMI, blood pressure, glucose, and cholesterol. Residents were also incentivized to visit again at the six and twelve-month time frames to measure any changes to their baseline results.

- Invite the new move-in to Urban Edge to meet members of the team and feel part of the community. In addition to incentivizing residents to visit the Family Van, Urban Edge hosted quarterly evening events for new residents that staff and volunteers from the Family Van attended. At each event, new move-ins were provided with health screenings and the health impact questionnaire was administered.

- Reconcile health impact questionnaires between the Family Van and Urban Edge. This took place to ensure that the data was being accurately recorded. Urban Edge staff would administer the survey and input the data into an online survey platform. Once the data was recorded, it was kept secured and only experts at the Family Van had access to the information.

This two-year pilot program offered a unique opportunity to learn by collaborating with a prominent health partner who has expertise in the community we serve. The plan we crafted was our best attempt to collect academic data that could further prove the impact that our affordable housing, coupled with services that address the social determinants of health, have on residents.

Lessons Learned

Throughout this pilot, we had to modify the program as we learned more about the ways residents respond. One of the first major lessons learned was how to coordinate the new resident move-ins. We had thought that it would be best to meet the resident while they were signing the lease for their new apartment. We quickly learned that the time of lease signing is extremely busy, with management documents and instructions about lease compliance, and that talk of a welcome visit and health programming did not make sense. It took follow-up from community engagement and property management to determine the best time to reach residents. Most often, the ideal time for new residents to meet was after working hours or during the weekend. Scheduling welcome orientations outside of standard 9:00 a.m.–5:00 p.m. working hours caused the staff time dedicated to this pilot to increase far beyond what was originally planned.

We know the Family Van offers valuable health services, and in survey data we collected 92 percent of Urban Edge residents said that someone in their family or other community members would utilize the Family Van's services if offered in convenient locations. While I believe that the location of the regularly scheduled van stations is convenient to most Urban Edge properties, convincing new move-ins to visit the Family Van was more challenging than expected. The program began by offering residents two movie passes to visit the Family Van for their baseline health screening. After a few months passed without any new residents visiting the Family Van, we increased the incentive to a $50 gift card. Still, the majority of residents who received health screenings did so through events at Urban Edge, and not by visiting the mobile clinic as originally designed.

In an attempt to understand the reason fewer than expected participants visited the Family Van, we analyzed HIQ data and preliminary findings of the biometric data. What we found was that of all fifty-nine residents who visited the van or received on-site health screenings, 92 percent have health insurance. We also found that of all new move-ins during this time period, 86 percent reported that they rarely or never have trouble paying for medical care or medication.

We began this journey with the thought that healthcare access was likely an issue for residents in the community. Not because we had any data that proved this, but because healthcare access had been widely talked about in our community for years. The data did not agree, and we learned that our residents were receiving healthcare at locations across the city, and the majority of our residents are insured with the highest percentage of people insured by MassHealth, Massachusetts's health program that combines Medicaid and Children's Health Insurance Program.

Overall, data was collected from new Urban Edge residents who moved in between January 2016 and June 2017. After completing data analysis, there was an observed improvement in self-rated health, safety, and stress. Residents reported feeling safer since moving into Urban Edge properties, they felt less stress than they did in their previous living situation, and they felt healthier overall.

What we learned confirmed what many already knew: quality affordable housing combined with quality services led to residents who feel safer, have less stress, and who are ultimately healthier. We also confirmed that relationship building is the key to success. Forming strong relationships between the Community Engagement team and new residents is essential to recruitment and crucial in follow-up.

Still, we had been left wondering: Was this the nexus? Did we need to literally bring health services to residents, or have we been contributing to positive health outcomes all along? For years Urban Edge has provided quality affordable housing, and over the past decade we have worked to hone our service offerings in financial coaching, benefits enrollment, leadership development, and access to resources. If our experience shows us that Urban Edge residents are not having trouble accessing care due to lack of insurance or location of health services, is there a better way for a community-based housing provider to contribute to improved health outcomes?

Health and Housing 3.0: Strengthening Partnerships and Integration of Services

Our work developing a new move-in program with the Family Van taught us that Urban Edge has been addressing upstream health factors for years through our programs and services, as well as through the built environment. It became clear that through our work in public safety, social supports, civic engagement, youth employment, among others, we had been helping people with short-term interventions that ultimately prevent health issues from arising later.

Data we collected showed that residents receive their care from nearby local health centers as well as from large hospitals. This prompted us to do more data collection, and in doing this we learned that out of the more than 2,800 residents who live in Urban Edge properties, 650 chose to receive their healthcare from a local health center that offers comprehensive health services, the Dimock Center (Dimock). After initial conversations with the executive team at Dimock, it was clear that we both shared similar visions and had the goal of cultivating a culture of health that will lead to a more equitable community.

The opportunity to work bidirectionally seems like a great opportunity. Urban Edge can identify residents who may need health services. The Dimock Center can utilize Urban Edge when their patients need additional supports, such as eviction prevention or financial coaching services. Recognizing our similarities and distinctions, we decided to put a plan in place to better serve Urban Edge residents.

Together we created a system where we focused on increasing the skills of the Urban Edge Community Engagement team by offering a formal training on addressing the social determinants of health as well as educating Urban Edge about all the services that Dimock offers. In addition to Dimock training the Community Engagement team, Urban

Edge informed Dimock's executive team about all the upstream services that Urban Edge offers its residents.

The Community Engagement team makes connections with residents during various moments in people's lives. Residents may provide us with insight into their life while participating in financial coaching or explaining why they are having tensions with a neighbor. During these moments, it is likely that a member of the Community Engagement team may have a window into the life of a resident that a medical doctor cannot see. It is during these moments where Community Engagement staff can identify issues that pertain to behavioral health, social isolation, safety concerns, or other stressors that, when identified early, can be helpful in addressing larger health issues.

It is because of this new understanding of our work that we began to design a streamlined referral system in the hopes of integrating our housing and resident services into a system that works synergistically with the health services offered by Dimock. By doing this, we believe we can improve the experience Urban Edge residents have when visiting their local health center (Dimock). We also believe this partnership will encourage residents to visit their health center more often. And if they knew about newer services that were offered at Dimock, such as dental and optometry services, more members of the family would visit the health center as well.

Together, Dimock and Urban Edge designed this partnership to better serve our residents and to promote improved health outcomes by addressing upstream drivers of poor health such as housing instability and food insecurity. By working together to increase a sense of community, and by providing a better consumer experience through an integrated referral system with follow-up, we believe that we can improve individual and community health.

The core elements of our program include the following:

- Joint training opportunities to better educate staff of Urban Edge and Dimock about relevant services, and to develop a more thorough understanding of the social determinants of health.

- Referrals from Urban Edge's Community Engagement team to Dimock in real time when encountering a resident who may need services offered by Dimock.

- Biweekly meetings to track referrals and determine if residents have been connected to the desired service.

The flow that was outlined consisted of six easy steps.

1. After a member of the Community Engagement team identifies a resident who has expressed interest in visiting Dimock for health services, a referral intake form is completed and the resident signs a waiver allowing both organizations to share information.

2. The Community Engagement team emails the referral form and signed a waiver to an email address specifically set up for this program. The email goes directly to a member of Dimock's executive team.

3. Dimock processes the referral form and contacts the resident within seventy-two hours.

4. The person who is referred to the case contacts Urban Edge to update us on the status of the referral. Common responses include "could not reach resident," "appointment scheduling," "no show to the appointment," etc.

5. If a resident is unable to make their appointment, the Community Engagement team contacts the resident to better understand what the barrier to receiving care was; that information is then relayed to Dimock and a new appointment is scheduled.

6.   Once a resident completes their health visit the Community
     Engagement team administers a quality-improvement question-
     naire to measure the level of satisfaction the resident has with his
     or her experience.

The purpose of both teams—Dimock and Urban Edge—meeting
biweekly is to make sure the aforementioned process is being followed
and to make sure that any resident having trouble connecting to care, is
connected with a warm handoff.

In 2018 we were able to connect fifty-four residents with the Dimock
Center.

The top services received at Dimock include:

- Optometry
- Dental
- Adult medicine, followed by pediatric services.

Top barriers to accessing healthcare (specifically appointments made at
Dimock) include:

- Time (job-related)
- Unexpected circumstance
- Childcare
- Questions about costs

The Dimock Center and Urban Edge have been neighbors for nearly
forty-five years; the two organizations are 0.3 miles away, door-to-door.
Naturally, we serve the same community and many of the same residents. However, the need to formalize our partnership became clear as
the relationship between housing and health has become a more widely
understood subject.

Not only did we connect residents to needed health services in a location that is conveniently located to their homes, we learned more about the

social determinants of health and how we, a community-based housing organization, can prevent future health issues. This pilot cemented a strong relationship between Dimock and Urban Edge and also inspired us to increase our knowledge about the social determinants of health. This experience made us realize how much more impact we can have if the entire seven-person Community Engagement team received more robust training.

Health and Housing 3.1: Sharpening the Saw

Today, three out of seven Community Engagement team members are now trained as community health workers (CHW). The rest of the team is scheduled to receive their training within the next year. This training is overseen by the Massachusetts Department of Public Health and run by the Boston Public Health Commission. The CHW training is an eighty-hour program that is based around ten core competencies:

1. Outreach methods and strategies
2. Individual and community assessment
3. Effective communication
4. Cultural responsiveness and mediation
5. Education to promote healthy behavior change
6. Care coordination and system navigation
7. Use of public health concepts and approaches
8. Advocacy and community-capacity building
9. Documentation
10. Professional skills and conduct

As our evolution into health and housing continues, we have learned more about the opportunity we have to impact the health of our residents. Now we aim to do this by helping residents live in stable housing, increase their sense of community, and create healthcare accessibility.

At Our Core: Developing Housing and Community

Urban Edge has been adding to Boston's affordable housing stock for decades. Over the course of forty years, we have added deed-restricted affordable units to the city, as well as preserved units that might have otherwise become too expensive for lower-income residents to afford. In forty-five years, we have added over 1,300 units of affordable housing to the community. And in 2015 we began working to add forty-nine more units of affordable housing in Boston.

We recognize that forty-nine units is only a drop in the bucket compared to the demand; however, we know that these units will present invaluable opportunities to the individuals and families who will live in these homes.

Creating Healthier, More Equitable Communities

The process to build these forty-nine units took several years. We had to acquire land, lead a community-engagement process, get local approval to build, apply for funding, then get through construction. This is a process that takes several years and finally, in early 2019, the new units were completed and families were moved in.

The people moving in now have the opportunity to live in a community that is interconnected and built with health in mind. Dimock will be part of the onboarding process as we welcome residents to their new homes. Taking the lessons learned from previous pilots we are now ready to move beyond the pilot and strengthen our existing partnerships with continual data collection and program refinement.

Have We Succeeded?

Has Urban Edge achieved improved population health, well-being, and equity? Not yet. We have expanded our understanding of how our housing and services impact health. We have also refined our suite of programs and services to better fit the needs of our residents. Urban Edge will continue to build housing with an intentional health focus that will one day allow all residents to lead healthier lives in equitable communities.

References

Carlson, S., and B. Keith-Jennings. 2018. "SNAP Is Linked with Improved Nutritional Outcomes and Lower Health Care Costs." Center on Budget and Policy Priorities, January 17, 2018. https://www.cbpp.org/sites/default/files/atoms/files/1–17-18fa.pdf.

Walsh, M., F. Doyle, and M. Valdes Lupi. 2018. *Health of Boston, 2016–2017*. http://www.bphc.org/healthdata/health-of-boston-report/Documents/_HOB_16–17_FINAL_SINGLE%20PAGES.pdf.

Chapter 9

Building Collaboration for Community Health

Lina Svedin
University of Utah

Building collaboration is not easy. Even in communities that are close-knit, uniting people around a common purpose and keeping them together can be hard. It is also, frequently, essential for change.

In chapter 4, Tina Tamai brings home the lesson that developing a collaborative network "requires intentional relationship-building." To build cohesion you need a thoughtful and deliberate process that helps the members of a group find their common purpose, goals, values, and capacity. That process, Tamai says, "Is not willy-nilly," but rather requires careful assessment of members' value base to ensure alignment. If the values, missions, the level of commitment and styles of working are too far apart, the network and its activities will be in peril. Culling an emerging network to a stable core with similarly driven and committed members may be necessary to really let the network form its identity and take root. Adding members who are not as aligned later in the network-building process may be less disruptive as a gelled core to the network can more easily accommodate differences without losing trust in the viability of the network or the vision it has established. The process of vetting members, surfacing values, and checking alignment also itself "helps foster a group mindset," which will make the group efforts more impactful.

This final chapter brings together several of the key lessons learned by and among the health leaders who have shared work and experience in the preceding chapters. While many teams faced challenges that seemed too daunting to tackle and many had to go back to the drawing board more than once, the collective experience in the preceding chapters proves that it can be done. This chapter highlights change leadership in practice, taking action while contributing to the communities that make change possible. The leaders that have been working for health in communities show significant growth over time, as community partners, advocates, and policy leaders. Their experience serves as a road map to navigate the challenges of community-engaged work and succeed in leading change from within communities.

Winning Minds: Solutions Have to Fit Into and Make Sense within an Organizational Culture

Change leaders motivate and create community buy-in by fitting "interventions" or solutions to the logic that makes sense to the community group. The idea has to fit with the conception the community members have of who they are and what their job is (Lin 2002). As a community health leader, if you can make sense of healthy solutions within the context of how people perceive and understand their role, their responsibility, and their organizational or professional culture, then they can make the solution their own. If they make it their own, and if they own it, then they can and will make endless variations of it to fit their everyday needs and the needs of their community members.

Emily Jackson had this very experience as she introduced Growing Minds to teachers in other schools, then to preschool educators, then to nutrition professors and students at universities and colleges, and eventually to doctors and nurses. When Jackson began her work in education, her background as a teacher enabled her to speak to the pressing interests of other teachers, to connect personally with them. Being able to relate new ideas and knowledge to community members in a language that they themselves use, and placing the new idea into the picture and understanding that the community has of its core values and mission wins hearts and minds.

Urban Edge works to provide high-quality affordable housing in an otherwise unaffordable city. While there is a long wait for families who want to access Urban Edge housing, the organization's goal is to make sure residents stay "housing stable" once they do get access. The services that the organization provides to prospective residents, families on the waitlist to get into Urban Edge housing, focus on making people housing stable, financially capable, and able to actively lead in their own lives. A person is considered housing stable when he or she can afford rent and do not feel at risk of being evicted. It is not just about staying housed, but about the opportunity to live stably and prosper. Because these are core values and goals that drive Urban Edge, the Robert Wood Johnson Foundation's culture of health framework was easy to map onto the organization's existing services and practices. The pathways to stability and prosperity frequently have to do with addressing underlying chronic health conditions and generational conditions of poverty and violence. The culture of health framework is now steering Urban Edge to focus more on improving health, well-being, and equity.

When Urban Edge developed its five-year strategic plan in the mid-2000s, the organization took a community-engaged approach.

The planning process involved residents, staff, and other community stakeholders, and through this engagement came the clear message that groups wanted this supportive housing organization to prioritize health and education in its work and mission. From the community conversations health was reported to be a key driver in what will strengthen individual residents, families, and, by extension, the whole community. Health was declared a shared value officially, and this charged Urban Edge to start changing course "to begin an evolution that would set our mindset and expectations about how we, as a community-based organization, can better impact the health of our residents through our housing and services." Along with prioritizing health in service provision, education was identified as an area that residents wanted more help with. The staff, residents, and community stakeholders jointly recognized that if low-income families have affordable housing, they can and will spend more of their time and resources addressing their health and educational needs. Not only did the culture of health framework map well onto Urban Edge's core values and goals, when the organization chose to do community-engaged strategic planning it became clear that these values were shared by key stakeholder groups and that residents themselves wanted support and focus on positive social determinants of health, including education. Charged with a clear desire for wellness and becoming self-supporting, Urban Edge started a number of new services. In the end, Urban Edge's collaborations with health professionals and using the culture of health framework taught them a lot about their resident community and their own work, and these things allowed them to grow.

In chapter 3, Michael Howard described how Madisonville, Kentucky, is a town with potential. Some may see it as a coal mining town that has lost its purpose and is on life support, but it has many of the things that allow a community to prosper. Whereas the coal and the mining companies used to be the economic engine of the town, the hospital system that was established to meet local needs is now the economic driver in the town and nearby areas. The town attracted quite a few educated professionals in the early 1940s and 1950s, and many of their families still live in Madisonville. Philanthropy is an important value among those who have stayed.

Howard is not coming up with new revolutionary ideas, but he is applying what we know works to the context of Madisonville and its available resources, starting with the hospital. "Most of what we are going for has already been tried in other places and has been shown to be effective in improving health for individuals and families. There is no need to re-invent the wheel. The medical center in Madisonville may be unusual in size and capability, but like most medical centers everywhere in the United States, we aren't doing it right. We still largely wait for people to get sick and then take care of them when they come to us."

"Doing it right" means addressing the root causes of illness and poor health, and those are not typically or even primarily genetic or microbial—they are social and economic. Social determinants of health make up 80 percent of what contributes to good or poor health. What Howard is proposing instead, which takes more effort but a lot less money, is a coordinated resource response to the social determinants of health that keep families dysfunctional, and, as a consequence, sick.

Rather than spending resources taking care of the symptoms of poverty and substance use disorder in families, Howard builds and leads coalitions of service providers (for-profit, nonprofit, governmental) in the collaborative effort to direct resources toward families whose members would otherwise frequent emergency rooms. It has worked in other settings, it is working in Madisonville, and it is cheaper for everyone than treating manifested illnesses. As a healthcare coordinator and coalition member Howard is reaching out to rural community members where they are most likely to show up outside their homes: at church and at barbershops. They are introducing conversations about health and health screenings—for example, encouraging blood pressure checks—to raise awareness of health, health resources, and to increase prevention of illness manifestation.

What the network is working at now involves getting those stakeholders with knowledge about the root causes—school nurses, social workers, teachers, and religious leaders—to connect dysfunctional families with community resources, maybe even a healthcare coordinator who can click them into a better-coordinated system of resources. The endgame involves helping individuals and families become functional, so they can take care of themselves and their children preventatively. However, the network also strives to make communities more health aware, health knowledgeable, and connected to resources, so the zip code in which a child is born ceases to be the primary predictor of their health outcomes over a lifetime.

In Hawaii, it has become apparent that having clarity of vision and purpose is important for group cohesion and sustainability. "Without a clear idea of the end goal and purpose of the group, the group will flounder and eventually fall apart. It also helps maintain trust and respect among members because each person understands their role and the end goal better." This lesson emerged over iterations, spurts of growth, and deepening, of the effort that today is called the Hawaii Good Food Alliance. At critical points in the Alliance's growth, the members had to pause and take stock of its mission again. There is a complex set of issues, beliefs, and values that are tied to food, not just in Hawaii but elsewhere, and the issue complexity along with a fluctuating number of network members forced the core group to examine and define the mission again and again. It even became necessary to narrow the scope of what the Alliance wanted to accomplish, to make the goals more tailored and narrower, to make sure the joint effort was effective and had greater impact on its intended targets. The core group ultimately decided this was more important than "trying to address a diverse array of issues and concerns among a wide audience of partners." The network of partners that remained and formed the Hawaii Good Food Alliance recommitted to supporting community leaders in their efforts to build "community-based food system networks to improve access and healthy eating among low-income populations." Fostering and supporting these grassroots networks and linking them together in larger and larger chains, the Alliance decided, was the best way to bring about a larger cohesive initiative that could bring about large-scale social transformation in Hawaii.

What the narrowing of scope and purpose of change networks in Hawaii illustrates is that change that is sought has to make sense in the context of the organizations and communities that will need to take action. The narrowing and redefining of goals and vision brought with it a natural streamlining of membership in the network that in turn made the network more cohesive and powerful. In order to grow a culture of health in a community struggling with health, both the understanding of the problem and the solution has to be synchronized with how participants view themselves and their situation.

Winning Hearts: Personal Connections to the Issue and the Solution Creates Advocates

Personal connections to the issues at hand, it turns out, are as important as the logic that connects professional frames and goals to health solutions.

The personal connection can transform a professional with access to large parts of the community or key stakeholder groups, from a participant to an advocate and a champion. And you are going to need champions if you are going to build solutions into the community, replicate successes, and make them sustainable.

Emily Jackson of Growing Minds did this by raising the respect and care for key professional groups such as school cafeteria nutritional staff, early childhood educators, and professors who had some interest in healthy food or locally grown food.

In chapter 7, DeWayne Barton discussed how he accomplished this with the neighborhood Peace Garden and with the Hood Tours. He created a space where members of the community could commune, play safely, and build connections. Young people in the community were proud of the Peace Garden and what it meant for the community, so they maintained it and kept it clean. Barton brought forward the rich history of the neighborhood, through his own actions—giving tours, getting a bus to take people through the neighborhood, and educating them about the neighborhood's past and cultural highlights. He embodied value and interest in the community to its members and to outsiders—lending additional validation to a history and a cultural richness previously unknown to most of the neighborhood residents.

Barton's commitment to community health is also deeply personal. As a child he would visit family in Asheville to get away from the busy lifestyle in Washington, DC. Asheville seemed like a warm and safe haven when DC was increasingly being taken over by drugs and street crime. After growing up and spending time in the navy, Barton moved back to Asheville, only to find that the neighborhood he remembered so fondly was being taken over by open-air drug trade, with garbage and used needles stacking up everywhere. The violence and hopelessness that the Burton Street neighborhood was displaying had Barton fearing that Asheville would go the very way that Washington, DC, already had. Along with infrastructure and job opportunities, the health of the community in black Asheville was being destroyed. He looked around "at mountains of discarded needles, homemade crack pipes, forty-ounce bottles, cans, lighters, and piles of garbage" and felt like he had to do something, so he started picking up the trash.

In chapter 6, Riana E. Anderson shares what brought her to the work she is doing with African American families to find ways to help their kids become more resilient in the face of racism. Studying clinical psychology as a graduate student Anderson ran into endless statements in books and articles about the difficulties in raising black children. Her experience had been quite different growing up. She had been raised by a loving, supportive, and culturally affirming family in Detroit, Michigan. Anderson was struggling to see examples in her own experience reflected in the studies she read. She eventually found studies with families like the one she had grown up with, but the vast majority of the research in the clinical psychology field was very deficit focused. They often focused on what was wrong with black families and how to fix them with some intervention. Anderson's commitment to her own research grew out of this juxtaposition. She has been determined to increase accessibility and representation of voices in the field of intervention research ever since. Even though her own commitment was firm, Anderson found something she never expected: "I never thought in a million years that I would have a team of people who *also* cared about the vision that I laid out" (emphasis mine). Anderson experienced the gratitude that comes from getting to work together with others who are passionate about important issues, and this is the food that nourishes great health leaders.

Education Needs to Include Kids and Adults

Children need to be educated about how to live healthier, healthier lives than their parents, but the adults need to be taught too. Without adults on your side buying into the ideas or solutions you bring to the community, then you are not going to have as much impact on the children.

In chapter 2, Emily Jackson examined how she learned this with parents, other educators, and other professionals. Many of them were just as in the dark about how food is grown and what the farms that grow the food they eat are like. Helping adults make the connection to local food, skill-building (cooking), and transporting them out of the school kitchen to the actual farms was a powerful tool to grow organizational and professional support for the program.

In chapter 7, DeWayne Barton discussed how he realized this in a different way as he was working with youth in juvenile hall trying to figure out how to teach them leadership skills that would translate into better safety and health outcomes in the neighborhood. While the work with youth in detention was worthwhile on an individual level, the lack of support from the administration charged with overseeing these youth was detrimental to the actual success of the training. There was a need for buy-in from the adults around these young people in order for the leadership education to take hold and be effective. The lack of apparent buy-in drove Barton to pursue other avenues to grow and rebuild his community.

Building From the Ground Up

There is a real need to involve those who are affected by a health problem or health equity issue from the beginning. One of the first and primary lessons in building the Hawaii Good Food Alliance was that the most effective solutions come from people who are on the ground. Tamai's recognition is that you should involve those affected in the process of solving the problems they face, regardless of whether that is in "identifying issues or developing solutions, it is essential to involve and trust people on the ground and in the community." Her experience is that the person who lives with the situation, "knows what the issues are and what solutions will work." There is also a deeper commitment in community-engaged change processes that is about showing respect and sensitivity to the situation. This approach, as Tamai and other authors showcase in this volume, leads to appropriate solutions. These are solutions that help the community in a way that the community wants to be helped, rather than fixes crafted and imposed by someone who does not know, or disregards, the community's wishes. Appropriate solutions generate community buy-in and support community efficacy. Not only do community-engaged change processes involve showing respect for the people involved but they also lead to better solutions that will reach more people in the community. Finally, community buy-in, efficacy, and trust are key elements to effectively engaging people in collaboration and to creating the synergy needed for social change.

Nampa, Idaho, had a similar experience, outlined in chapter 5. The Nampa team recognized that they needed to have the youth whose health the group was planning for involved and present. In addition to youth and the network of community health stakeholders, the group also saw the need to engage leaders and influencers from the start. The leadership team in Nampa also recognized that "there are often mixed reviews about including funders at the planning level" when you are trying to produce community change. In Nampa's case, however, bringing funders to the table from the start "was highly beneficial, because it allowed for honest dialogue, two-way communication, a better understanding of expectations from the grantor and grantee, and another set of expertise to provide insight." As a result, the Nampa team was able to adjust its funding priorities in a way that meet the foundation specifications and expectations and thereby secured funding for the youth health project.

In black Asheville, urban renewal led to a thirty-year war on drugs. In the Burton Street neighborhood this war led to mass incarceration of black youth, and the overall health of the community was interrupted. The great reputation and connection of the community were lost. DeWayne Barton grappled with the following question: how does a community rebuild itself from the inside out? When the City of Asheville wanted to close down the neighborhood community center, Barton and the community group "convinced the youth to get involved working to help save the center to start writing letters, and even a song, to the city, state, and federal officials." Their efforts paid off, and the city backed off on closing the center. Together, these members of the Burton Street community continued to clean up and renovate the community center.

Being privy to conditions and personal stories of those in the youth detention center, Barton came to realize that the community was really the cradle of learning for these young men and women. The schools the youth came from were not teaching them anything; they were merely detaining them for a certain amount of hours per day. Where the students were learning was in their neighborhood, in their community, and they were taking the skills they learned there to school "to practice what they're taught at home and in the neighborhood." Barton was in a position between his work in the evenings with the Burton Street community and his daytime job at the YDC "to clearly see the connection between lack of support and poor infrastructure and how that led to an increased number of young people going to prison." Having realized this, Barton left his day job at the YDC to instead "focus on the neighborhood with renewed efforts." He and his wife started paying youth to pick up trash, and they established the Peace Gardens with the goal "to establish infrastructure and relationships that would allow health-related programs to occur."

Over the years, the Burton Street Peace Gardens have become "a sanctuary for positive action, designed to create neighborhood food security, community cohesion, and a vibrant, sustainable local economy." Based on the clean-up and community development work Barton and the community had done, Asheville was awarded a federal Weed and Seed grant. Unfortunately, only 30 percent of the grant money went to the neighborhood itself.

Building from the ground up also increases the sustainability of the efforts that community leaders initiate. In black Asheville, the effort to build from the ground up and building sustainability in culture of health initiatives included specifically young people, for young people to improve the physical environment of the community in an environmentally informed way. This included "a plan to be able to train young people in trade skills that were environmentally friendly." Barton enlisted people "who knew about solar, weatherization, and building in an environmentally conscious way." Because there were no prior training programs that would teach "young people in green skills that would be focused in their neighborhoods," Barton set out to create Green Opportunities (GO).

In his own youth, Barton had been through a training program of the kind that he was establishing. With Green Opportunities, Barton had the idea that they would "make the neighborhood the school itself." The goal Barton envisioned was "for the kids to advance from obtaining their GEDs to establishing trade skills, and then go on to become entrepreneurs or inventors, or to seek advancement in school." He saw a lot of creativity in these young people that had not been tapped in any way. In addition,

Barton saw the need to "engage with workers and business leaders in the community," thereby creating a sustainable and productive collaboration.

Start with the Smallest Unit and Build from That

The authors in this volume make absolutely clear the possibility of starting change with small steps, right where you are standing now. Howard states that in order to save rural America it will not take a miracle, "It's just a matter of will and resources. And a little time." Jackson, on growing health in Appalachia, states in chapter 2: "You just need a little land … seeds, plants, water … easy, peasy." For all the hardship and destruction that his community has faced, Barton states this most plainly in chapter 7: "If you really want to build a healthy and flourishing environment for your community, start with picking up trash and building a garden."

Reflecting on what got him started, Barton stated that one morning, a short time after he had returned to Asheville, he stepped outside and ended up between two men shooting at each other. At what he describes as a profoundly sobering moment, he decided that he needed to try and help restore the health of his community. Looking around the neighborhood he saw giant piles of garbage everywhere and "decided to start by simply picking up trash."

Let's not teach our children, the next generation, and our fellow community members that making a difference requires money and elaborate constructs because then they are never going to try. That message is disempowering and leads to inaction, disconnection, and despair. We see plenty of evidence in these chapters that small changes can be powerful. Starting from the ground up is how you build most things sustainably. The message for change should be start where you are, use what you have, share freely with others, and it will be enough.

Relationships Are Key

There are many individuals, groups, and organizations that are doing excellent work stretching already thin resources; many people get what they need today so they can get by and, in a very real sense, live to fight another day. But in order to make better use of the resources communities have, and to address deeper causes and conditions of poor health, we need to collectively look at the problem/situation jointly. We need to pool knowledge, resources, and effort so we can leverage what we have and problem solve more intelligently so that we can get to the root causes that drive how people live, work, and play in unhealthy ways. We are, in a very real sense, better together. When an individual gets their underlying and fundamental needs met, they get better. When they get better, families get better. When families get better, they contribute more to their communities. When people contribute more to their communities the world gets better.

One of the lessons from the Hawaii Good Food Alliance was that "maintaining a high standard of values sustains morale and the sense of integrity needed to promote commitment and sustainability. Over time, whether members stay committed, relationships are kept, and the organization/cause is sustained, depends on complete authenticity and sincerity."

In chapter 5, Jean Mutchie and Shannon McGuire state that Nampa's transformative experience has not been an easy one, but, they argue, it has been extremely worthwhile. One of the lessons from this community leadership team was the need to be willing and ready to have hard conversations. Once tensions rose in relation to specific solutions, there was a natural tendency to want to pull away and avoid having that conversation. Having an experienced facilitator to help the group through those tough situations was extremely helpful. It helped each partner voice their concerns and opinions but also their desires for change to continue. While it became clear in this process that conflicts needed to be dealt with quickly and effectively, it also became clear that out of the conflict rose more sustainable solutions that benefitted the community.

Conflict is inherent to any attempted change—when something old is being shaken up, moved, or thrown out for something new, different, or unfamiliar—that creates conflict. Trying to get people to move in one direction and not another creates conflict. Thus, how conflict is managed is key. If conflict is managed well, all parties can be better off and have their needs met in the new situation.

Another example of lessons learned about the importance of building relationships was at Urban Edge. Energized and empowered to help residents improve their health and well-being, the supportive housing organization set up a pilot with a local university to bring a mobile healthcare unit, the Family Van, to Urban Edge housing complexes. The Family Van was established to do initial health screenings for new residents and to provide some medical treatment. New residents were incentivized to go to the van for their health screenings, medical needs, or medical referrals. After a few months, when none of the new residents had visited the van, Urban Edge and the healthcare partner increased the incentives for residents, but still hardly anyone utilized the service. This led Urban Edge to ask residents about their healthcare coverage and where they would go to receive medical care if they needed it. They found that they had mistakenly assumed that residents did not have access to healthcare when, in fact, most of them had health insurance coverage and were utilizing a community health clinic right next door to Urban Edge. With a better understanding of their residents' healthcare assets and needs, Urban Edge revamped its efforts to support health by developing a partnership with the community clinic they had lived next door to for decades. Through this two-way partnership residents were better supported and nonresident patients at the health clinic gained access to supportive services provided by Urban Edge.

Growing Loose Community Collaboratives into Strong Advocacy Alliances

Several of the stories conveyed in these chapters show how individuals and groups can go from being caring, hard-working, and collaborative, to becoming tight-knit, effective, and committed community advocates.

The Hawaii Good Food Task Force is a great example of this. The task force asked a highly regarded facilitation team, Islander Institute, to conduct a meeting with the Food Network. The feedback they got from the facilitators was to reexamine the group membership in order to align their purpose and goals. As a consequence, the membership was narrowed to community leaders who were doing one core thing; developing food distribution systems that connected production to the community and served low-income populations. The remaining group members were able to retreat, bond, and increase their shared commitment, and they started "working on a charter of agreed values and goals, resulting in a focused and well-articulated purpose statement" that aligned "membership and staying targeted on a specific mission and agreed-upon strategies is an imperative." The network of networks had successfully transitioned and grown into a dedicated and focused group of network builders and advocates. The group even chose the word *alliance* to signify their commitment to taking an activist-advocate role.

What DeWayne Barton is doing now—after years of organizing, cleaning up, and creating opportunities for the next generation in the Burton Street community—is educating people about what the neighborhood is like. He is building a larger community with a passion for Burton Street's history and culture by running Hood Tours and publishing the *Hood Huggers Green Book*.

Barton saw the value of connecting the community with its history and out of that grew inspiration for the future. There are things about the history of a community that can serve as a touchstone of strength, pride, cohesion, and culture. The eradication of that history and the disconnection from that history can also serve as a drain on communities. When tour buses flew through the black neighborhoods, Barton asked how these communities were being portrayed by the tour companies. In order to find out, he visited the Asheville Chamber of Commerce that told him that there was no real interest in black history. Rather than having the established tour companies distribute a flier about black history in the area, which they offered to do, Barton decided that he would lead—he would tell the story of the neighborhoods himself. He actively connected the history of place and people, his neighborhood, and his people to the state of health in the community today, bringing insight but also encouragement for the future.

The Hood Tours support other organizations that are working to save and restore historic places in the neighborhood. Barton is building forward, leading by example, and helping others do the same. Barton states that his idea for the *Hood Huggers Green Book* "is loosely modeled after the *Negro Motorist Green Book*." With the *Hood Huggers Green Book*, Hood Tours wants "to show people where and how to connect today, right now, with black-owned businesses." During the tours, Barton "take[s] my visitors to the Peace Garden to wander through the vegetables, the flowers, and the sculptures to soak in the serenity and creativity that emanates from that wonderful space." This is literally and figuratively growing a new prosperous and historically informed future for black Asheville, leading by example, starting new collaborations, and supporting the community in moving into a culture of health.

Managing the process of bringing networks together is critical to collaboration. Sometimes referred to as backbone individuals, these network leaders can play a pivotal role in keeping the group meeting, making sure that meetings are run efficiently so no one feels like their time is wasted, and encouraging partners to keep showing up to meetings. Facilitating face-to-face interactions are essential for building trust, exchanging challenges, and best practices, as well as facilitating resource sharing when needed. While teleconferencing can meet the needs of dispersed groups, it seems like face-to-face meetings are where the magic happens, where collaborative networks can bond and grow into strong advocacy coalitions.

Networking can be effective in addressing "monumental, complex problems where conventional, linear strategies and interventions are ineffective." Conventional funders do not readily accommodate the growth and change aspect of network collaboration. There needs to be enough coordination as a task and enough infrastructure funded "to enable networks to survive long enough to begin implementing change strategies." In dynamic relationship structures, such as an evolving collaborative network without the necessary support infrastructure, "burnout is inevitable." The Hawaii Good Food Alliance "found networks to be valuable as they enable intersection, cross-pollination of ideas and resources, as well as cross-organizational collaboration, which can transcend geographical and sector boundaries and mobilize synergy with greater magnitude to create social change." However, it was also clear that difficult decisions needed to be made about network participation, and enough task and coordination support was pivotal for the network's survival.

In Nampa, Idaho, the team leaders learned how to leverage collaboration and partnership into new productive ventures. They also show just how key personal relationships are to successful collaboration. Once the issue of child obesity in Nampa became a focus and grant money became available to make innovative and transformational change, these community health leaders activated potential advocates.

Leading for Change

These culture of health leaders are addressing persistent and serious community health issues and the conditions that lead to poor health outcomes. They are surveying, discussing, and dialoging with communities about their experiences and the community's priorities. This is how they are building community-based solutions to health-related issues that the community cares about. This volume is full of examples of how communities, when asked and resourced, are able to share deep knowledge about what works in their community and how to build resilience. It is pivotal to recognize that in order to build a culture of health in the United States and in communities everywhere, we need to respect and honor the experience of members of those communities we want to engage with.

Positive change is possible and is supported by driving a desire for change, pushing ourselves, those around us, and communities out of complacency (e.g., Kotter 1996). You have to care, have passion, and take initiative to start change. Having a vision of what could be or how things can be different, is important, as is communicating that vision often and to the many people you encounter. Any time you try to change something you are pushing up against something. You are inevitably trying to move something else out of the way—a system, a power distribution, a privilege—to make room for a new idea. Therefore, expecting and managing conflict is an important component of change management. The trick is not to let the obstacles stop the work of trying to move in a new direction or to introduce a new idea or set of expectations. Change is boosted by early wins and small victories that help envision bigger wins up ahead. These aspects of building a culture of health in communities can and are currently manifested through leadership, by the chapter authors who are leading from within their communities.

What is equally evident and central is that leadership requires followership. Change only happens through people, and if we are serious about respecting the communities where we seek change, change needs to come through leadership with communities in the direction they themselves value. There are just as many examples of the successful engagement of communities, stakeholder groups, and organizations in this volume as there are instances of leadership. As leadership gains followership there is a relationship-building that will support all of the transitions, visions, and actions that it will take to bring about community change. Many of the communities that have the worst health outcomes are also communities with a long history of adversity, structurally and institutionally reinforced by leaders who did not listen to them, by decisions made in rooms where they did not have a voice. Trust, as a result, is scarce. It is absolutely essential that moves toward improving health and reducing barriers to health come with an understanding of the existing state of trust. Trust is built by doing trustworthy things; by aligning words with action and acting consistently over time leaders can be the touchstone of trust that communities need to come together. Collaboration and altruism can flourish in communities with trust—it is the growing ground for social capital. With social capital, health leaders have an infrastructure on which to build sustainable change. Leading this kind of change, together with others who are also passionate and committed, is what makes great culture of health leadership. The authors in this volume show it is possible. Let's go out and lead from within for a more equitable and healthier America in every community.

References

Kotter, J. P. 1996. *Leading Change*. Cambridge, MA: Harvard Business School Press.
Lin, A. C. 2002. *Reform in the Making: The Implementation of Social Policy in Prison*. Princeton, NJ: Princeton University Press.

Bios

Volume Editor Bio

Lina Svedin, PhD, is an associate professor in the Department of Political Science at the University of Utah. Lina is Swedish by origin and has worked both as an area specialist for the Swedish national government, and as a research leader and training director at the Swedish National Center for Crisis Research and Training. A majority of her research has focused on governance challenges in crisis conditions including ethics and accountability in the distribution and management of societal risk. Much of her current research focuses on taboo topics in public policy, including homelessness, suicide, child sexual abuse and economic inequality, and the impact of policy on marginalized populations. Dr. Svedin teaches administrative theory, policy analysis, program evaluation, ethics for public administrators, as well as governance and the economy in the Master of Public Policy and the Master of Public Administration programs. Dr. Svedin was part of the first cohort of the Interdisciplinary Research Leaders fellowship with the Robert Wood Johnson Foundation and is currently on an Intergovernmental Personnel Act assignment to the School of Advanced Air and Space Studies at Air University, Maxwell AFB. Prior to this assignment, she was the Director of Public Affairs Programs, College of Social and Behavioral Science at the University of Utah.

Contributor Bios

Chapter 1: Leading from Within: Creating a Culture of Health through Leadership and Community-Grown Solutions

Lina Svedin (see above bio)

Chapter 2: Cultivating Health in Appalachia

Emily Jackson directs Appalachian Sustainable Agriculture Project's Growing Minds program and proudly serves as a Robert Wood Johnson Foundation Culture of Health Leader. She lives in the beautiful mountains of western North Carolina with her husband, one dog, two cats, and a varying amount of chickens. Emily believes deeply that every child should have the opportunity to grow a garden.

Chapter 3: Saving Rural America, Starting with One Girl

Michael Howard is the founder and CEO of the ARCH Community Health Coalition. He spent eleven years in the US Army reserve, and has been a biomedical researcher, biology professor, healthcare executive, and nonprofit leader. He has a BS in biology and a PhD in physiology and biophysics.

Chapter 4: Network Strategies and Cross-Collaboration to Strengthen Community Food Systems

Tina Tamai, MPH, JD, began networking communities as program manager at the Hawaii Department of Health. Success in generating cohesion and collaboration among community food systems leaders led to the founding of the Hawaii Good Food Alliance, a statewide network dedicated to improving food access and healthy eating among disadvantaged populations.

Chapter 5: One Community, Two Voices

Shannon McGuire is the Chief Empowerment Officer at Spark Strategic Solutions. Outside of the office you'll find her rallying to improve the local food system, empowering teens as future leaders, and exploring the wonders of nature with her family.

Jean Mutchie is the West Treasure Valley community health manager for St. Luke's Health System. She co-chairs the Nampa Healthy Impact Coalition and is a current Robert Wood Johnson Foundation Culture of Health Leaders fellow. During her twenty years in the healthcare industry, her work has focused on community health and health equity initiatives that impact children.

Chapter 6: EMBRacing Community-Engaged Research: Engaging, Managing, and Bonding through Race Intervention

Monique C. McKenny is a graduate student researcher at the University of Miami in the School of Education and Human Development. She studies how racial discrimination relates to both psychological and physiological health outcomes for black youth and how racial socialization practices may serve a protective function for black families.

Riana Elyse Anderson, PhD, is an assistant professor in the Department of Health Behavior and Health Education at the University of Michigan's School of Public Health. She completed her PhD in clinical and community psychology at the University of Virginia, a clinical and community psychology doctoral internship at Yale University's School of Medicine, and a postdoctoral fellowship in applied psychology at the University of Pennsylvania.

Chapter 7: Rebuilding Affriclachia

DeWayne Barton, founder and CEO of Hood Huggers International, is native to Asheville, North Carolina, and is a Gulf War veteran. A local artist with national recognition, Barton serves on the NC Arts Council Board and is a Robert Wood Johnson Culture of Health Leader. Barton co-founded Burton Street Peace Gardens and Green Opportunities.

Chapter 8: The Evolution of Health and Housing for One Community-Based Organization

Robert Torres, MPA, is the Director of Community Benefits at Beth Israel Deaconess Medical Center in Boston, Massachusetts, where his work focuses on investing in programs and services that address the social determinants of health in historically underserved communities. He has spent the last decade working in the areas of affordable housing and mental health and substance use policy.

Chapter 9: Building Collaboration for Community Health

Lina Svedin (see above bio)

Acknowledgments

This is the second volume in the series "Interdisciplinary Community-Engaged Research for Health." The series is guided by an insightful group of community-engaged researchers and community partners serving as an advisory board: Andriana Aribiotes, Kathleen Call, Jennifer Malat, Kristen Kalsem, and Sherrie Flynt-Wallington. Each of these outstanding scholars and community leaders works tirelessly to promote community-engaged research. I would also like to thank Elizabeth Scarpelli at the University of Cincinnati Press, who has gotten as excited about the prospect of a series like this as Farrah Jacquez and I are. Her ability to think big is such an inspiration and source of encouragement.

I am so grateful for the reviewers who took time from their own ventures to carefully read and provide feedback on the chapters in this volume: Sarah Shepard, Daniel Chapman, Glen Mays, Fran Feltner, Julie Metos, Robert Forbis, Juliet Carlisle, Sharon Mastracci, Christopher Jensen, Andrew Jackmauh, Ashley Lewis, Becky Utz, Kristy Cottrel, Erin Moore, and Lara Bauer.

I would also like to thank the Robert Wood Johnson Foundation (RWJF) for the considerable investment they are making to create a culture of health in the United States. Through four programs, Clinical Scholars, Healthy Policy Scholars, Culture of Health Leaders, and Interdisciplinary Research Leaders, RWJF is cultivating leaders who are changing the landscape of health outcomes in the United States.

Furthermore, the chapter authors and the work featured in this volume would not have come together and been introduced to this larger audience without the access, support, and training provided by the Culture of Health Leaders program. For the vast majority of the contributors, this is the first time they're seeing their own words, work, and passion in print. I am tremendously excited about the ripples, the inspiration, and the empowerment that can come from these change leaders sharing their experience, strength, and hope. I'm grateful to each and every one of the authors for trusting me with their time, and their stories, and for jumping on the opportunity to put this book together even though this was new to most of them.

I would like to thank the public affairs programs staff at the University of Utah for patiently and lovingly putting up with me as director. Victoria Medina, Beth Henke, Erin Moore, and Lara Bauer, you are the best team I have ever worked in. Thank you for all you do, for me and countless others.

Finally, I would like to express my sincere gratitude to Air University for the opportunity to land in a new stimulating context as a visiting professor and the vote of confidence to add to the Air Force curriculum and thinking. The change in pace, care, and support that I have enjoyed since I arrived has allowed me to wrap up many backlogged projects that were begging to get out the door, including this volume. And a joyous thank you to my colleagues at the School of Advanced Air and Space Studies, who have made the transition such a treat and spiritually uplifting.

Lina Svedin
Maxwell Air Force Base
Montgomery, Alabama, July 2019

Index

A

AB Technical College, 122

academic achievement, 87–89, 93, 122

action research. *see* community-engaged
  research

adults

  barriers to volunteering, 41

  and farm-to-school involvement, 16, 19,
    23–26, 158

  health problems among, 36, 76, 88, 144

  rally to save Asheville community
    center, 116

Affrilachia (black Asheville). *see* North
  Carolina, Asheville

African-American children and families.
  see EMBRace; North Carolina,
  Asheville

Albuquerque, New Mexico, 59

alcohol abuse, 88

Anderson, Riana

  implementation of EMBRace, 11, 86–87,
    90, 93–94, 99–100, 102–3, 104, 157

  intervention developer of Racial
    Empowerment Collaborative,
    85–86, 102–3, 104

anxiety, 88

Appalachian State University, 22, 123

Appalachian Sustainable Agriculture
  Project (ASAP)

  becomes southeast regional lead agency,
    18

  challenges USDA over school nutrition
    services, 18

  Growing Minds Farm to School
    program, 15, 17–20, 22–24

Growing Minds @ University (GM@U),
    21–22, 24

  integrates farm to school into
    curriculum, 16–22, 25–26

  marketing problems between schools
    and farmers, 25

  and partnership with Head Start, 20–21

  receives grant from Kellogg
    Foundation, 17–18

  trains chefs, 20

  works with local distributors, 26–27

arcades, 98

Arthur R. Edington Education and Career
  Center, 122

ASAP. *see* Appalachian Sustainable
  Agriculture Project

assisted living, 130

asthma, 76

automation, 34

B

backbone individuals, 167

Baraka Community Wellness, 133–34

barber shops, 44, 154

Barton, DeWayne

  designs community accountability plan,
    123

  founds Green Opportunities, 11, 112,
    120–23, 161

  founds Hood Huggers and Hood
    Tours, 126, 156, 166

  founds Peace Garden, 11, 156, 161, 162,
    166

  involvement with Youth Development
    Center (YDC), 116, 158, 160–61

Barton, DeWayne *(cont.)*
    president of Burton Street Community
        Association, 122
    removes trash from neighborhood, 11,
        157, 161, 162
    and restores black Asheville, 11
Barton, Safi, 11, 117, 119
beauty shops, 44
benefits screening and enrollment, 136,
    137, 140
Big Island (Hawaii), 55–59
bituminous coal, 32
black Asheville (Affrilachia), 11
black history, 126–27, 166
Black Parenting Strengths and Strategies
    (BPSS), 90
blood pressure checks, 154
Blue Cross of Idaho Foundation for
    Health, 68, 71, 73
Blue Ridge Community College, 22
Blue Zones project, 56
Boise State University. Initiative for
    Healthy Schools, 72
Boston, Massachusetts
    affordable housing in, 11–12, 130
    hosts New Entry Community Food
        Systems Conference (2017), 59
Boston Public Health Commission, 145
box truck, 78
BPSS. *see* Black Parenting Strengths and
    Strategies
burnout, 65
Burton Street. *see* North Carolina,
    Asheville
bus tour companies, 126, 166

C
cafeteria staff, 18, 24, 156
cafeteria taste tests, 19, 20, 22, 25, 26

calculate, locate, communicate, breathe,
    and exhale (CLC-BE), 92
cancer, 36
CAP. *see* community accountability plan
    (CAP)
cardiovascular disease, 88
CBPR (community-based participatory
    research). *see* community-engaged
    research
CDC. *see* Centers for Disease Control and
    Prevention
census tracts, 10, 68, 69, 75–76
Center for Medicare and Medicaid
    Services (CMS), 38
Centers for Disease Control and
    Prevention (CDC), 50
change
    barriers to, 9
    conflict inherent in, 164
    factors for creating successful, 8–9, 65,
        169
    impact of insurance upon, 38
    and networking, 61, 65, 167
    starting with small steps, 162
chefs
    Chefs Move to Schools programs, 20
    Junior Chef competition program in
        Hawaii, 53, 55
Children's Health Insurance Program
    (Massachusetts), 140
churches
    role in raising awareness of health
        issues, 44, 154
    weatherizing, 121
CHW. *see* community health workers
citizenship activities, 41
civic clubs, 44
civic engagement. *see* community-engaged
    research

CLC-BE. *see* calculate, locate, communicate, breathe, and exhale
clinical trials, 6
CMS. *see* Center for Medicare and Medicaid Services
coalition building, 30, 38, 43–44
coal mining, 31–32, 34–35, 152–53
CoHL. *see* Culture of Health Leaders Program
collaboration
  importance of, for health equity, 9
  and networking, 65, 167
  trust essential for, 169
  varying degrees of, in community-academic partnerships, 7
  see also specific partnerships
collective impact theory, 53–54
"comeback lines," 91
communication, 64–65
community-academic partnerships, 6–7
  see also specific partnerships
community accountability plan (CAP), 122, 123–25
community-based participatory research (CBPR). *see* community-engaged research
community-engaged research, 2, 6–9
  see also specific partnerships
community health coordinator, 46
community health workers (CHW), 145
Community Supported Agriculture (CSA), 19, 24, 55
compassion fatigue, 9
conflict, 164
consultants, 74
consumer engagement. *see* community-engaged research
cooking demonstrations, 17, 19, 22, 25, 52, 54, 55, 134, 158
Cooperative Extension agents, 19–20

coordinating entity, 63
County Health Rankings and Roadmaps, 2–3
crack cocaine, 111
Crossroads Resource Center, 58
CSA. *see* Community Supported Agriculture
CTSA. *see* National Institutes of Health. Clinical and Translational Science Award
Culture of Health Leaders Program (CoHL). Robert Wood Johnson Foundation, 2–4
  see also specific partnerships

D
daycare workers, 20–21
dental services, 142, 144
depression, 88
diabetes, 36, 76
dietitians, 19, 22, 79
Dimock Center, 141–45, 146
disabled population, 75
DNA (song), 87
Double Up Food Bucks program, 53, 54
drug abuse, 111, 113, 116, 119, 157, 160
Duke University. World Food Policy Center, 22

E
early childhood educators, 20, 156
Electronic Benefit Transfer (EBT), 52–53, 54, 55
EMBRace (Engaging, Managing, and Bonding through Race)
  communicating with stakeholders, 99–101
  community partnerships, 97–101
  developing and implementing, 86, 91–93

EMBRace *(cont.)*
  and engaging in community research,
    101–5
  interventions to reduce racial stress,
    86–87, 89–104
  lessons learned, 96–97, 99, 101
  purpose of, 11
  research process for, 93–95
  staff and training for, 95–96, 102–5
employment
  benefits of, 4–5
  in Madisonville, Kentucky, 34–35
  in Nampa, Idaho, 69–70
  for youth, 141
Empowerment Resource Center of
    Asheville, 122
energy audits, 121
entitlement spending, 70
eviction prevention, 136

F
facilitators, 59, 63, 64, 81, 163, 165
faith-based community gardens, 78
Families First, 133
family trees, 92
Family Van, 135–39, 141, 164
farmers and farmers' markets
  EBT access for, 52–55
  education and training for, 57
  role in farm-to-school program, 15–27
farm-to-school movement
  classroom cooking demonstrations, 17,
    19, 22, 25
  farm field trips, 16, 17, 19, 22, 24, 25, 26
  funding for, 17–18, 19, 23–24
  Growing Minds Farm to School, 15–20
  and Growing Minds @ University,
    21–22, 24
  integrating into curriculum, 16–22,
    25–26

  interesting rural adults and children in,
    23
  now available in all 50 states, 27
  partnership with Head Start, 20–21
  and university professors, 19, 24, 151, 156
  working with local distributors, 26–27
Federal Emergency Management Agency
    (FEMA), 75, 79
fee-for-service model of sick care, 36, 38
financial coaching, 136, 137, 140
fitness equipment, 72–73, 81
floodplains, 75, 79
Florida, 18
FLS Energy, 121
Food Basket, 55
food deserts, 55, 69, 75
food pantries, 69, 77, 78
Food Stamp Nutrition Education. *see*
    Supplemental Nutrition Assistance
    Program (SNAP)
fruit consumption, 10, 50, 52, 55–56
funding
  for Asheville, North Carolina projects,
    112, 119, 122, 127, 161
  for EMBRace project, 104
  for farm-to-school programs, 17–18, 19,
    23–24
  and funder involvement, 83, 159–60
  by Hawaii DOH, 54
  for Hawaii Good Food Network, 58–60
  for Healthy Impact Nampa Coalition,
    68, 77
  High Five Community Transformation
    Grant, 71–73, 80, 82
  lack of, in community-engaged
    research, 8
  mini grants for farm-to-school
    program, 19
  need for community participation in
    awarding, 7–8

not accommodating for network
    collaboration, 167
RWJF Culture of Health Leaders
    fellowships, 3–4
RWJF Invest Health grant to Nampa,
    Idaho, 73

G
gardens
    faith-based community, 78
    in farm-to-school movement, 15–20, 22,
        23, 25–26, 52, 54
    Peace Garden, 11, 112, 117–20, 122, 127,
        156, 161, 166
Georgia, 18
GM@U. see Growing Minds @ University
GO Kitchen (Green Opportunities), 122
Great Recession, 70
Green, Victor, 126
greenhouses, 54
Green Opportunities (GO), 11, 112,
    120–23, 161
grocery stores, 69, 78
Growing Minds Farm to School program
    Jackson initiates, 15–20
    Jackson's work with key professional
        groups, 20, 156
    lessons learned, 22–27
    relationship with ASAP, 18–19
    training chefs, 20
Growing Minds @ University (GM@U),
    21–22, 24

H
Hawaii (Big Island), 55–59
Hawaii Department of Health (DOH),
    47–48, 50–51, 54, 56
"Hawaii Food for All" (report), 58–59
Hawaii Good Food Alliance
    beginning of networks, 54–57

building network of networks, 10, 48,
    49–50, 154–55, 167
core values, 62–65, 163
need for community representation,
    61–62, 159
network transitions to Hawaii Good
    Food Task Force, 57–59
pilot programs, 50–54
restructuring network of networks
    framework, 59–60, 165
vision for future, 60
Hawaii Good Food Network, 10
    funding for, 58–60
    transitions to Hawaii Good Food
        Alliance, 60, 165
Hawaii Good Food Task Force, 10, 57–59,
    165
Hawaii Island Food Alliance, 56
Hawaii State Department of Human
    Services (DHS), 52
Head Start, 20–21
health care
    barriers to accessing, 144
    disparities in, 10–11
    impact of racial discrimination upon,
        87–88
    as key driver in community health, 152
    trends in, 37–38
    types of insurance, 38
health fairs, 44
health impact questionnaire (HIQ), 135,
    137–38, 144
health insurance
    impact upon visits to Family Van, 139
    people lacking, 38, 76
    as result of employment, 4, 33
    types of, 38
health screenings, 164
"Healthy Eating in Practice" (2018
    conference), 22

Healthy Impact Nampa Coalition, 68, 77
heart disease, 36
High Five Community Transformation
      Grant, 71–73, 80, 82
high school students
   graduation rates, 75
   participation in Traveling Table Mobile
      Food Pantry, 69, 78
highway construction, 115, 122, 131
HIQ. *see* health impact questionnaire
Hispanic population, 73, 75
homelessness, 80
Hood Huggers Green Book, 127, 166
Hood Huggers International, 111–12, 123,
      126–27
Hood Tours, 126–27, 156, 166
Hopkins County, Kentucky, 36
housing
   affordable, 11–12, 77, 80, 129–31,
      135–38, 140, 146
   discrimination in, 129
   effect upon health outcomes, 129, 135
   first-time home buyer classes, 136
   home ownership, 69–70, 75
"housing stable," 132, 151
Howard, Michael, 10, 152, 162

I
I-95 highway, 131
Idaho, Ada County, 71
Idaho, Nampa
   census tracts in, 10, 68, 69, 75–76
   childhood obesity in, 10–11, 71–72, 76,
      168
   demographics, 69–71, 73
   Food Access Committee, 77
   funders' involvement at planning level,
      159–60
   lessons learned, 80–84, 163
   local government, 69, 70, 71, 73, 77, 82

McGuire's collaboration with mayor,
      69, 73
Nampa Chamber of Commerce, 71
Nampa Healthy Conditions
      Assessment, 75–77, 81
Nampa Healthy Kids Coalition, 72, 73
Nampa School District, 71
youth involvement, 81, 159
Idaho, Treasure Valley, 10–11, 70, 76
Idaho Department of Health and Welfare,
      71
Idaho Foodbank, 78
inertia (fear of change), 31
intervention research. *see* EMBRace
Islander Institute, 59, 165

J
Jackson, Emily
   on children's disconnect from food
      source, 9–10, 23
   founds Growing Minds Farm to School
      program, 15–20, 22–24, 25–27, 162
   founds Growing Minds @ University,
      21–22, 24
   on need for adult involvement in
      farm-to-school movement, 16, 158
   partners with Head Start, 20–21
   raises respect for early childhood
      educators, 20, 156
jobs training. *see* trade skills
journaling, 91
JumpStart, 133
Junior Chefs program, 53, 55

K
Kalihi Palama Health Center, 51–54
Kentucky.
   farm-to-school movement in, 18
   Madisonville, decline of coal mining in,
      31–32, 34–35, 152–53

Madisonville, healthcare in, 10, 29–31, 32–34, 36–37
opioid epidemic in, 37
Kohala Center, 55
Kokua Kalihi Valley Comprehensive Family Services (KKV), 51–54, 58–59

L
Lamar, Kendrick, 87
Latino population, 73, 75
LBT Collaborative. see Live Better Together Collaborative
leadership development, 136, 140
legislative support for community-engaged research, 9
Lenoir-Rhyne University, 22
Leroy, Dan, 121
lesson plans for farm-to-school curriculum, 19
lifespan in U. S., 37
lignite, 32
listening, 12
listserv, 100
Live Better Together Collaborative (LBT Collaborative), 53, 55, 56
logo, 53
Louie Family Foundation, 60

M
machinery (in coal industry), 34
Madisonville. see Kentucky
mapping exercise, 136
Massachusetts Department of Public Health, 145
Massachusetts House of Representatives, 131
MassHealth, 140
McGuire, Shannon, 10–11, 69, 73–74, 163
McKenny, Monique, 11, 85–87, 90–91
McKinney-Vento Act, 80

Medicaid, 72, 140
memorandum of agreement (MOA), 97–99
Meter, Ken, 58
Miami, University of, School of Education and Human Development, 90
Michigan, University of. School of Public Health, 90
middle schools, 41, 97
MOA. see memorandum of agreement
mobile clinics. see Family Van
Molokai, 56
Mountain Bizworks, 122
movie passes, 137, 139
MS Lean Landscaping, 112
Mullen, Dwight, 124
Mutchie, Jean, 10–11, 70, 163

N
Nampa. see Idaho, Nampa
National Association for the Advancement of Colored People (NAACP), 103, 115
National Farm to School Network, 15–18
National Institutes of Health (NIH)
on benefits of community-engaged research, 7
Clinical and Translational Science Award (CTSA), 8
National School Lunch Program, 18
NC Farm to Preschool Network, 21
Negro Motorist Green Book (Green), 127, 166
network of networks
beginning of model, 54–57
effectiveness of networking, 167
networking defined, 65
re-structuring framework, 59–60
Tamai on, 10, 149, 159
theory of change, 65
transition to community framework, 57–59

neural connections, 21
New Deal Works Progress
    Administration, 33
New Entry Community Food Systems
    Conference (2017), 59
newsletters, 100
newspapers, 44, 115
New York City, 130
NIH. *see* National Institutes of Health
North Carolina, Asheville
    Asheville Chamber of Commerce, 126,
        166
    Asheville City Council, 121–22
    Asheville Design Center, 123
    Asheville Housing Authority, 121, 122
    black history in, 126, 166
    Burton Street Advisory Committee, 115
    Burton Street Community Association,
        122
    community accountability plan, 123–25
    credit unions in, 125
    designated as an environmental justice
        community, 123
    deterioration of neighborhood, 113–14,
        156–57
    effect of highway construction upon,
        116
    Green Opportunities project, 11, 112,
        120–23, 161
    Hood Huggers and Hood Tours,
        111–12, 123, 126–27, 156, 166
    mass incarceration of black youth, 160
    Peace Garden, 11, 112, 117–20, 122, 127,
        156, 161, 166
    Pearson founds Burton Street, 115
    rally to save community center, 116, 160
    receives Weed and Seed grant, 119, 161
    referred to as "Affrilachia," 11
    Youth Development Center (YDC),
        116–17

North Carolina, University of
    Asheville, 120, 124
    Chapel Hill Center for Health
        Promotion and Disease
        Prevention, 22
North Carolina Child and Adult Food
    Program, 21
    see also Appalachian Sustainable
        Agriculture Project (ASAP);
        Growing Minds Farm to School
        program
North Carolina Department of
    Transportation, 122–23
nutrition
    school nutrition staff and education,
        16–21, 26–27, 52, 55, 57, 156
    USDA nutrition services, 18, 47–48,
        50–51
    see also Supplemental Nutrition
        Assistance Program (SNAP)

O
Oahu, 56
Obama, Michelle, 20
obesity
    adult, 36, 76
    childhood, 10–11, 36, 71–72, 76, 168
    as major public health issue in U. S., 50
opioid-related overdoses, 37
optometry services, 142, 144

P
participatory action research. *see*
    community-engaged research
patient-centered medical home (PCMH),
    38
Patient-Centered Outcomes Research
    Institute (PCORI)., 8
payroll, 35
PCMH. *see* patient-centered medical home

PCORI. *see* Patient-Centered Outcomes
    Research Institute
Peace Garden, 11, 112, 117–20, 122, 127,
    156, 161, 162, 166
Pearson, E. W., 115, 126
peat, 32
pediatric services, 144
Pennsylvania, University of. Racial
    Empowerment Collaborative, 85–86,
    95, 102–3, 104
pharmacies, 78
Philadelphia, Pennsylvania. *see* EMBRace
phone conferences, 56
physical inactivity, 36
physicians
    influence in healthy eating, 22
    in Madisonville, Kentucky, 33
PLAAY Preventing Long-Term Anger
    and Aggression in Youth. *see*
    Preventing Long-Term Anger and
    Aggression in Youth
policy, systems, and environmental (PSE)
    approaches, 72
potluck dinners, 52
poverty
    census tracts' identification of, 75–76
    correlation with poor health, 10–11, 37,
        40, 42, 151, 153
preschools & pre-K readiness, 18, 21, 22,
    25, 27, 133, 151
prescriptions, 78
Preventing Long-Term Anger and
    Aggression in Youth (PLAAY), 90
primary care delivery models, 38
Prison Books, 117
private insurance, 38
produce distributors, 27
PSE. *see* policy, systems, and environmen-
    tal approaches
public housing, 121

public insurance, 38
pulmonary disease, 36

Q
questionnaires. *see* surveys and
    questionnaires

R
race
    discrimination and effect upon
        academic achievement, 87–89, 93,
        122
    and influence on local public policy, 124
    racial discrimination and effect upon
        health, 87–88
    racial socialization, 88–92
    racial stress and trauma, 11, 91
Racial Empowerment Collaborative
    Anderson as intervention developer at,
        85–86, 102–3, 104
    McKenny as program coordinator, 86,
        104
    Stevenson as leader of, 95, 102, 104
Racial Encounter, Coping, Appraisal, and
    Socialization Theory (RECAST),
    89–90
radio ads, 53
real estate speculation, 131
RECAST. *see* Racial Encounter, Coping,
    Appraisal, and Socialization Theory
recipes, 52, 79
redlining, 129, 131
referral systems, 142–43, 164
relationship building, 64, 140
Republican party, 70
restaurants, black-owned, 98, 127
Robert Wood Johnson Foundation
    (RWJF)
    culture of health framework and Urban
        Edge, 132, 151, 152

Robert Wood Johnson Foundation *(cont.)*
    Culture of Health Leaders Program
        (CoHL), 2–4
    Invest Health grant awarded to
        Nampa, Idaho, 73
    support for Hawaii Good Food
        Network, 58–59
role playing, 92
rural communities
    Appalachian Sustainable Agriculture
        Project, 9–10
    farm-to-school movement, 15–27
    health disparities in, 10, 29–46
    inferiority complex in, 31
RWJF. *see* Robert Wood Johnson
    Foundation

S
safety net programs, 21
San Francisco, 130
schools
    breakfast and lunch programs, 41
    gardens in farm-to-school project,
        15–20, 22, 23, 25–26, 52, 54
    middle, 97–99
    nutrition staff and education, 16–21,
        26–27, 52, 55, 57, 156
Science, Technology, Engineering, and
    Math. *see* STEM
sculpture park, 118
seeds, 19
segregation, 132
Self Help Credit Union, 125
service learning, 40
Shelton Farms, 24
shuttles, 78
Silicon Valley, 130
Simone, Nina, 126
sleep deprivation, 88

smartphone rewards app, 134
smoking, 36, 37
SNAP. *see* Supplemental Nutrition
    Assistance Program
social capital, 169
social media
    to disseminate information about health
        care, 44
    for EMBRace, 100
socioeconomic factors and healthcare, 37,
    40, 60, 80, 97, 105
South Carolina, 18
Spark!, 73
staff meetings, 24
stakeholders
    for coalition building in rural
        communities, 30, 47, 154
    to combat childhood obesity in Nampa,
        Idaho, 10–11, 71, 159
    communicating EMBRace goals and
        interventions, 99–101
    moving from participants to advocates
        and champions, 154–56
    need for different for community
        collaboration, 8–9
    for public health programming in
        Hawaii, 47
    for Urban Edge planning process, 132,
        151–52
St. Alphonsus Medical Center, 78
STEM (Science, Technology, Engineering,
    and Math), 41, 42
Stephens-Lee Alumni Association, 126
Stephens-Lee Community Center, 126
Stevenson, Howard
    co-develops EMBRace with Anderson,
        86, 93, 95, 102–3
    leader of Racial Empowerment
        Collaborative, 95, 102, 104

St. Luke's Children's Hospital, 78
storytelling, 91, 92, 125
student loan counseling, 136
sub-bituminous coal, 32
substance use disorder (SUD), 39
Sundance Power Systems, 121
Supplemental Nutrition Assistance
        Program (SNAP)
    in Hawaii, 47, 50, 51, 52–53, 54, 55,
        57–59
    for Urban Edge participants, 136
    use in Nampa, Idaho, 75
surveys and questionnaires
    for Burton Street development, 123
    for EMBRace research, 92
    of farm-to-school programs, 18
    of Nampa community, 74, 76
    for Urban Edge participants, 133, 135,
        137–38, 144

T
"the talk," 89
Tamai, Tina, 10, 149, 159
taxes
    allocation of tax money, 70
    preparation of, 136
teachers
    assistance to STEM, 41
    and farm-to-school movement, 16, 17,
        19–21, 24–25, 151
    involvement in EMBRace, 94
    as stakeholders, 154
teleconferencing, 167
Tennessee, 18
Torres, Robert, 11–12
trade skills, 120–23, 161
train-the-trainer healthy cooking skills, 52
transportation, lack of options in, 10, 68,
        69, 75, 77–79
trash removal, 11, 114, 157, 161

Traveling Table Mobile Food Pantry, 69,
        78
Treasure Valley. see Idaho, Treasure Valley
Triangle Park, 126
Trover, Faull, 33
Trover, Loman, 33
Trover Clinic, 33
Turner, Lindsey, 72, 74

U
unemployment and under employment,
        4–5
Union Capital Boston, 133–34
university students and professors, 19, 156
    assistance for STEM teachers, 40–41
    Growing Minds @University (GM@U),
        21–22, 24, 123, 151
    see also specific universities
Urban Edge Community Development
        Corporation
    assumptions about residents' health
        care, 139–40, 164–65
    Community Engagement team, 137,
        139–45
    community health workers (CHW),
        145–46
    developing affordable housing units,
        140, 146
    influence of RWJ Foundation upon,
        132, 151, 152
    move-in program coordination with
        Family Van, 135–39, 141, 164
    partnership with Dimock Center,
        141–45, 146
    provides educational programs for
        residents, 133–34
    purpose and mission of, 12–13, 129–32,
        147, 151
    strategic plan, 132–33, 151
urban renewal, 115, 160

U. S. Department of Agriculture (USDA)
    and conflict with farm-to-school
        movement, 18
    and conflict with Hawaii Department
        of Health, 47–48, 50–51

V
value-based healthcare, 38
vegetable consumption, 10, 50, 52, 55–56
vendors, 26
vouchers, 98

W
Wallace National Good Food Network
    (2018), 59
weatherization, 121, 161
websites
    County Health Rankings & Roadmaps,
        2
    for EMBRace, 100
    Growing Minds, 19
Weed and Seed grant, 119, 161
Western Carolina University, 21–22
Western North Carolina Green Building
    Council, 122
"What Works for Health," 3
"What Works for Health Disparity
    Rankings," 3

"What Works? Social and Economic
    Opportunities to Improve Health," 2
WHO. see World Health Organization
Wholesome Wave, 54
Winter Green, 121
W. K. Kellogg Foundation, 17–18
World Health Organization (WHO), 7

Y
YDC. see Youth Development Center
YMCA (Hawaii), 51–54
YMI Cultural Center, 126
youth and youth providers
    incarcerated youth, 116–17, 160
    rally to save Asheville community
        center, 116, 160
    represented in Nampa, 81, 159
    summer jobs for, 136
Youth Credit Union, 125
Youth Development Center (YDC),
    116–17
YWCA (Asheville), 122

Z
zip codes, 37, 154
zoning policies, 79